# THE

# PERFECT

# FIT DIET

D1364807

HOW TO LOSE WEIGHT, KEEP IT OFF,
AND STILL EAT THE FOODS YOU LOVE

# THE
# PERFECT
# FIT DIET

## LISA SANDERS, M.D.

St. Martin's Griffin ≈ New York

www.stmartins.com

Library of Congress Cataloging-in-Publication Data

Sanders, Lisa, 1956–
    The perfect fit diet : how to lose weight, keep it off, and still eat the foods
you love / Lisa Sanders.—1st St. Martin's Griffin ed.
        p.   cm.
    First U.S. ed. published in 2004 with subtitle: Combine what science
knows about weight loss with what you know about yourself.
    Includes bibliographical references (p. 365) and index (p. 379).
    ISBN 0-312-33823-6
    EAN 978-0-312-33823-7
    1. Reducing diets.   2. Food preferences.   I. Title.

RM222.2.S239 2006
613.2'5—dc22                                                      2004063284

First published in the United States by Rodale Inc.
First St. Martin's Griffin Edition: January 2006

10  9  8  7  6  5  4  3  2  1

For Tarpley and Yancey,
the best friends and daughters a mother could have

# CONTENTS

# ACKNOWLEDGMENTS

This book initially grew out of a research project I worked on with my friend and mentor, Dr. Dawn Bravata. Her warmth, intelligence, and discipline were a model for me throughout the research we did together on low-carb diets, right up to this revised version of the book.

I am also indebted to my sister Shelley, who shared with me the ups and downs of her personal struggle with her weight and let me share them in these pages. In addition, I could always count on my sisters Andrée and Leslie to help me keep my language and ideas tied to the world outside the doctor's office.

I am grateful to the patients who shared their stories with me. They have been my inspiration and education.

Josh Horwitz, of Living Planet Books, transformed my ideas into a book by believing in them and in me. Gail Ross, my agent, has been unflagging in her enthusiasm. My editor, Jennifer Weis, and publisher, Matthew Shear, have been generous with their vision and imagination, for which I am most grateful.

I must also thank Catherine Saint Louis, Katherine Bouton, Joel Lovell, Paul Tough, Ilena Silberman, and Dan Zalewski, my editors at *The New York Times Magazine*. Their skillful editing taught me much of what I know about writing and everything that I know about writing well.

I owe thanks to Dr. Julie Rosenbaum, my colleague at the Yale primary care residency program, and Valerie Duffy, a researcher and nutritionist at the Yale School of Medicine and the University of Connecticut. Each brought a careful scientific eye to the manuscript, saving me from all manner of embarrassment; whatever errors remain are mine alone. The meal plans were developed with the help of a marvelous dietitian, Marcie Garcia.

Thanks also to Tony Horwitz, Geraldine Brooks, and their dining room table, where so many ideas have been born. Dr. Dena Bravata and Dr. Anjali Jain provided their insight and frequent wisdom freely. Margaret Spillaine and Bruce Shapiro were ever ready to supply advice and comfort, as needed.

Steve Huot, the director of the Yale primary care residency program, encouraged my interest in obesity from its start and remains an essential support. Patrick O'Connor and David Coleman at Yale's Department of Internal Medicine made this book possible in many ways. Thank you. Thanks also to the staff of the Family Health Center: Dr. Henry Gift, Cindy Collette, and June Detlefsen. Their humor and balance continues to make going to work a pleasure. Ideas always need a stimulating environment in which to grow. My tiny plot has been generously enriched by many scientists, researchers, and friends who helped me bring this book to fruition. My thanks to Dr. Gretchen Berland; Dr. Laura Whitman; Dr. Eric Holmboe; Dr. Linda Bartoshuk; Dr. James G. Gibbs; Kelly Brownell, Ph.D.; Dr. Walter Kernan; and Dr. Ashgar Rastegar.

Thanks also to the friends who made this book possible in ways too many to be recounted: Richard Kreider, Lindsay Patterson, Jenny Brown, Ian Ayres, Louise DeCarrone, Neale and Steve Berkowitz. Also, Juanita Stallings, Terry Lavallee, Mark Gracia, Joe Gallagher, Lea Bowman, Janel Hackney, Hiram "Pat" Patterson, Sandra Karakoosh, Dwight Lopes, Melanie Smith, and Bonnie Erbe. You are the heart and soul of this book.

But finally, it is Jack to whom I owe this book. His wisdom, insight, intelligence, wit, and thoughtfulness shaped every idea, every page I have ever written. His love and devotion supported me from television, through medical school and residency, and finally to my work as a physician and writer. His kindness and empathy, his humor, and his incredible skills as an editor have enriched my life, my work, and, of course, this book.

# INTRODUCTION

How many times has this happened to you? You meet a friend you haven't seen in a while and she looks great! You gently inquire, and she nearly explodes with the answer: After years of trying one diet or the other, she has finally found the right one. It was there the whole time and now that she's on it, she can't imagine why she didn't see it before. It's so great, she says, and she gets to eat so many of the foods that she loves. She's never hungry, and she's losing weight like crazy. Before you know it, you're on it too.

Once you're there, though, it doesn't seem so great. These are not foods you want to eat. This is not the way you want to feel. You're not losing weight, just patience. You wonder what she was doing that you're not, why she feels so good and you don't. What's wrong with you?

There is nothing wrong with you, and there is nothing necessarily wrong with that diet. You didn't fail this diet; this diet failed you.

Why this is true represents a major shift in the way science is approaching all medicine and the issue of weight loss in particular: Each of us is different. What we're discovering is that not every treatment has the same effect on every patient. With weight control, that means that the regimen that works for one person may not work for another. In diets, as in so many things, one size does not fit all.

Unfortunately, when a doctor sees a patient who wants to lose weight, he doesn't ask, "What do you eat?" In fact, research suggests that he's much more likely to tell you what you *should* eat. It's the same diet he puts everyone on. He assumes, as so many of us have in the past, that for this one problem—being overweight—there is one cure, the diet he happens to prefer. And if you can't eat that way, then as far as he is concerned, you're *choosing* not to lose weight. You clearly are just not motivated enough.

Or maybe he just tells you to eat less and exercise more. Duh.

Chances are, you *would* eat less, if you knew how—if you knew the secret to consuming fewer calories without feeling hungry, tired, cranky.

This book is for people who know they are motivated enough but recognize that there are aspects of their diet that they can't seem to change. This book is for people who have tried to "eat less and exercise more" but can't figure out how. It's for people who want to eat in a sane and rational way that will make them feel good and be healthy—not only while they lose weight but for life. This book is for people who instinctively know that the claim of a magic bullet—the diet that works for everyone—is a myth, but they don't know how to figure out which diet might be right for them.

There is a truckload of science out there about diets—much of it from new and exciting research—investigating what we eat, why we eat it, what makes us full, and what makes us different from each other when it comes to how we eat. I've spent the past several years delving into that literature, sorting through the good research and the not-so-good, looking for connections and hidden truths. The most compelling conclusion I've reached is this: The deeper you dive into the science of weight loss, the more the solutions return to the medical, psychological, and lifestyle profile of each individual dieter. This book is designed to help you choose and customize a diet that fits you to a T—a diet that's a perfect fit because it's designed not for everyone but for you. A diet that will help you lose that extra weight, keep it off, and yet make room for the foods you really love—and can't give up.

The truth is that we are all on a diet. A diet is simply what you eat. And that diet either works for you—allowing you to achieve and maintain your target weight—or it doesn't. Based on the much-touted rise in obesity in this country, it's clear that most Americans are on a diet that doesn't work. My job and the job of this book is to help you find the diet that will work for you—not just for now but for a lifetime. That is the perfect fit diet for you.

# PART 1

# THE NEW SCIENCE OF WEIGHT LOSS

# CHAPTER 1

# THERE IS A PERFECT DIET FOR EVERYONE

Y OU ARE WHAT YOU eat."

You've heard it all your life. And it's true: What you eat can—quite literally—shape what you become. Our mothers told us this to get us to eat more good food and less junk food, and I believed mine, at least enough to get through the plate lined with fingers of fish and mounds of string beans, chased down with a cup of whole milk slowly warming in the jelly jar glass. This concept has been incorporated into our cultural identity (as American as apple pie) and advertising slogans (Wonder Bread: Builds stronger bodies in twelve ways) and the automatic truths we're taught in our health and nutrition classes from first grade on up.

But what about the other way around?

Would you also believe that "you eat what you are"? Yet, it's also true: What you eat is shaped by *who you are*. What you eat is, in fact, a direct reflection of you—genetically, culturally, psychologically, and environmentally. If that is true (and there is plenty of evidence that it is), then clearly the best diet to achieve and maintain good health and weight is going to be different for each of us.

That is the premise of this book.

I call this book *The Perfect Fit Diet,* but let me tell you a secret: There is no diet that is perfect for all of us. There is only the diet that is perfect for you. The diet that is right for you will not be the same diet that is just right for me or really for anyone else.

You already know this is true. Chances are, you have tried diets before this one and maybe something worked (for a while) or maybe it didn't work at all. But ultimately it wasn't the right diet for you—if it had been, you wouldn't be here today.

You see, we are all different. And that difference extends from the smallest part of us—our genes—to the more familiar selves we see in everyday life. Sure, we have much in common: We all have two arms and legs, two eyes, and one mouth. But despite these similarities, we don't all look the same. Our bodies don't work the same. Our minds don't think the same. Our lives have taken different shapes and paces. What we eat, how we eat, how the food we eat makes us feel, how that food is handled by the tiny chemistry sets inside our bodies—these are also quite different among individuals. How can we then expect there to be only one "right" way to eat? How could there be only one way to achieve and maintain our target weight? It's ridiculous. It's unrealistic. And yet this is how many of us think.

What will *your* perfect diet look like? Certainly it's got to be made up of foods you enjoy; it has be a diet that makes room for the foods you love—even the "bad" foods. It's got to be a way of eating that will give you the foods that trigger your sense of fullness and satisfaction. It should be a diet that allows you to eat until you are satisfied at mealtime and confident that you will be ready to eat by your next meal and not two hours before. It should be a diet that will offer you foods that maximize your metabolism and enhance your health. It should be a diet that will make you *feel* better, not just look better. Finally, the perfect diet is a diet you will be able to live with— for the rest of your life.

Research shows that the number-one predictor of a dieter's success is longevity—the longer you can stick with a diet, the more weight you will lose, the longer you will maintain that loss, and the healthier you will be. But for a diet to last a lifetime it has to feel good, and to feel good it has to fit. This book will guide you through five simple steps to help you find a diet that is perfect for you.

So, what are those steps?

First, you keep a diet diary. That's the hardest part of the whole process. But I'll walk you through it. And it will be one of the most valuable parts of this whole process.

Using that information, you fill out the Perfect Fit Questionnaire. Based on my own research, it is a detailed look at what you eat, how you eat, and how what you eat makes you feel. It asks about your health, your family, your lifestyle. Answering these eighty-three questions will give you a complete picture of the factors that will shape the perfect diet for you. Filling it out takes about an hour, but believe me—it's an hour well spent.

You score the questionnaire to find out which of three basic diet types might be right for you.

But you can't stop there.

Then, you use the questionnaire to customize your diet to fit your food preferences, your metabolism, your medical history, and your lifestyle.

Finally, you use the questionnaire to help you identify the attitudes and behaviors that have undermined all the diets you've tried in the past.

When you are done, you will have a way to eat that will help you finally achieve and maintain the weight you want. The three basic diets in this book are designed to help you lose up to 2 pounds a week for as long as you need to. Once you achieve that weight, your diet will help you maintain it for the rest of your life. Why will this diet last when none of the others have? Because this diet was designed for you. It was designed to fit you perfectly. It was built from the ground up to satisfy your taste buds, your stomach, and your body.

For a diet to succeed, it has to be easy enough to do the right thing. We make dozens of decisions each and every day that have some impact on our weight. Whether you are trying to lose weight or just struggling against the world that is determined to make us fat, most of those daily decisions have to go in the right direction. That means it has to be easier for us to do the right thing than the wrong thing. A perfect diet should be built around the dozens of decisions that make up your daily life. It has to take into consideration what you like to eat, when you like to eat, and how what you eat fits in with the rest of your life. In other words, it's got to fit you perfectly. The only way to get that fit is to shape a diet around you.

Throughout this book I will tell you about a few of the many dieters who have followed my program to find a diet that was perfect for them. Let me start with the story of Sarah. After decades of struggling against the accumulating pounds, she has finally found a way to achieve the weight loss she desired and a way to eat that will last a lifetime.

*The Perfect Fit for Sarah (lost 28 pounds)*
*Challenges always tickled my psyche—maybe it's part of the oldest-child profile—so when the triple whammy of thyroid disease, a slipped disc, and menopause piled over 30 pounds onto my size-6 frame, I attacked my weight gain with enthusiasm: Atkins, Weight Watchers, South Beach. I tried them all but failed. I became a "diet groupie," devouring every diet*

*and weight-loss magazine article, book, and Internet site seeking the magic answer. Some held that magic, I am sure, but not for me. I found my normally optimistic self spiraling toward apathy.*

*Friends and family encouraged me to just accept myself as I was and try to be happy. But how could I? Could I be happy lacking energy? Happy when my knees ached and my back protested the extra pounds? Happy staring at a stranger in the mirror? Fortunately my challenged inner voice rallied. And not long after I found* The Perfect Fit Diet.

*I admit that the frustrated, apathetic part of me sought a reason to justify just letting it collect dust on the shelf, but ultimately the "individualized approach" toward weight loss appealed to me. It made sense to me. When a spring shopping trip revealed yet another leap to a size 14, I finally started my diary.*

*Suddenly so much about my failures started to make sense to me. I was clearly a low-carb person, but it couldn't be just any low-carb diet—it had to be* my *low-carb diet. Atkins steaks and cheeseburgers held no allure. I replaced them with fish, nuts, and cheese. I couldn't live without fruit—or chocolate—so I didn't. Finding replacements for the sandwiches that I always ate for lunch was a challenge that was easily met.*

*In eight months I lost the weight I hated so much, that I couldn't reconcile myself to despite the support and encouragement of my good friends. And now I'm at a weight I thought I'd never see again and I'm back to a size 6 at last. I've lost the weight, but what's even more important, I've found a way to eat that I like and that likes me.*

## WHY WILLPOWER FAILS US

We like to think that a behavior as fundamental as choosing what we put in our mouths is well within the domain of human willpower—especially with the abundance and variety of foods available to us today. We can eat fruits and vegetables out of season and fish caught halfway around the world, and drink wine from grapes grown on virtually every continent. But there is also an aspect to what we eat that seems beyond our complete control.

We may exercise our mighty wills in choosing where, what, and when to eat, but we make those choices within a personal framework that is beyond choice. What foods we like or dislike, how we prepare them, why we want to eat in the first place, and why we feel full and satisfied at the end of a meal—all these aspects of eating are defined by our genetics, our culture, and our lifestyle. We rarely, if ever, think about them, yet they shape the world of eating within which we make our choices. As much as we would like to, we cannot simply will these deep-set characteristics into conformity with a list of healthy-eating principles we learned in high school and are exhorted to follow by our doctors and dieticians.

We can *decide* to get the fat out of our diet—but if we eat out everyday, we're not going to be able to do it. We can *decide* to give up snacking and eat only three meals a day, but if the foods we eat leave us hungry between meals, we're not going to be able to do it. We can *decide* to go on a diet that strictly forbids us to eat so many of the foods we love, but ultimately—and usually a lot sooner than that— we are not going to be able to do it.

So often, when we fail, we tell our friends and ourselves that we just don't have the willpower to diet. Well, none of us do—that's not how willpower works. Willpower is like an airbag—it is one of those extra tools we have to call on when life spins out of control. But you can't use it every day. You can't count on willpower for the days when work and traffic and family have your nerves as frazzled as the loose end of a nylon rope. You can't count on willpower on the days when you rush out of the house without breakfast and run around until the mid-afternoon when you have to go to a reception for a friend or colleague. For the daily encounters with food and desire you need a plan that takes into consideration what those daily needs will be like—where you eat, what you eat, when you eat. You have to have those essentials built into a diet if it's going to work for you.

In order to exercise real choice, we need to recognize the ways in which our bodies and our lives affect our decisions. To make realistic choices—choices you can really live with—you need to understand how they will work given who you are and how you live.

This is something we know and accept in most parts of our lives—we rarely waste our time and effort in "choosing" to make time stand still or the sun not set. We recognize that our choices must be made within the structure of a 24-hour day.

While few things in life are quite as unyielding to choice as time and the movement of the earth in its orbit, our values, our culture, even our lifestyle can seem just as difficult to change. Recognizing the framework in which our individual choices are made is key to making changes that work. Science is beginning to discover and define many of the aspects that shape our choices—how our genes, our upbringing, and our lifestyle create the structure in which our choices about diet are made. Once we understand those structures, we can make choices that fit us and our lives. Only then can we discover the diet that is perfect for us.

I know, I know: Change is hard. It's why so many of our New Year's resolutions are long forgotten by Groundhog Day, and why so many diets fail within days of beginning. We need, as the old prayer tells us, the courage to change what can be changed and the serenity to accept what we cannot. We also need a way to tell the difference. This book is designed to help make those distinctions—to identify those behaviors—and to guide us in the right direction.

## WHY I CREATED THE PERFECT FIT DIET

My education in the trials of weight management began years before I went to medical school. For decades I'd watched the collateral damage of failed dieting strategies at home, where my own family offered a telling example of the individual, and often elusive, nature of weight gain and loss.

My father's side of the family is overweight; my mother's side is thin. My older sister, Shelley, inherited my father's genes. Ever since childhood I've watched Shelley struggle with her weight. She's the classic yo-yo dieter. She goes on a diet, loses weight, but can't stick to the diet and ends up regaining all the weight—and often a little more. Over the years, she's tried every weight-loss fad on the market.

Every failure is accompanied by a cycle of self-loathing and depression, which often begins its own cycle of eating and a lapse in exercise. I love my sister, and it's been painful to watch this intelligent and self-aware woman struggle to manage her weight. When I hear doctors say it's a lack of willpower, I only have to think of Shelley to know it's not true.

Shelley is typical of the failed dieters I meet every day in my clinical practice. They see their lapses as moral failures, proof of their weak wills. But dieting isn't about moral strength—it's about compatibility between an individual and a chosen diet. It's about finding a diet that won't fail you when the crunch comes.

I'm writing this book to offer people like Shelley a way out of their cycle of guilt and shame by helping them find a weight-loss program they can live with. They need hard information—so many dieting "facts" are, in fact, fictions—and they need encouragement in tackling the very tough challenge of shedding weight in an environment rigged to make us gain.

My girlfriends, my patients, and anyone I meet who finds out that I'm a "diet doc" ask me the same question: Is there anything that actually works? These people have been beaten, both physically and psychologically, by a series of failed attempts at dieting. They are all looking for authoritative news about how to end the cycle of failed diets and finally succeed at weight control.

Science has finally offered us some hope. Using what researchers are discovering we are now able to design diet programs tailored to fit each dieter, as opposed to the one-size-fits-all approaches that have dominated the field for decades. Now that mainstream science is finally engaging nutrition and obesity as a serious field, we will be seeing more and more authoritative information about how our genes, our lifestyle, and our personal taste preferences affect our ability to control our weight.

*The Perfect Fit Diet* is every dieter's long-sought compass for navigating the thicket of competing diet claims, the rational path for the thinking person who wants to lose weight.

## A NEW LOOK AT WEIGHT LOSS

For the past several years, I've been working with a team of researchers at Yale and Stanford universities. We've conducted a systematic analysis of hundreds of weight-loss studies dating back to the turn of the twentieth century. Initially, we were looking at whether low-carbohydrate diets, such as the Atkins diet, are any better or worse than other types of diets. That study was published in *The Journal of the American Medical Association (JAMA)* in 2003. In the course of my research, I have read literally hundreds of studies on the effects of different diets on weight loss and other aspects of health. After years of sifting through these studies, I was struck by a surprising pattern that seemed to defy conventional medical wisdom: All these diets did work—for some people.

Time after time, a study would show that a diet worked dramatically for, say, 10, 20, or even 30 percent of the people who tried it while others lost little or no weight. How was it that nearly every diet had winners and losers? Each seemed to have a cadre of people for whom the diet worked wonders, while other dieters failed miserably.

I became intrigued by the possibility that there is no single diet that works for everyone but, rather, different diets that work for different people. Perhaps the key to weight loss is not the single best diet, or the most motivated person who is trying to lose weight—though clearly, diet and motivation are important. Perhaps the key lies in matching the right dieter to the right diet.

One of the conclusions of my research, and the research of many who came before, is that there are aspects of any diet that help predict how well it will work. For example, the lower the calorie content of the diet, the faster you will lose weight. And the longer the diet lasts, the more weight you will lose. But I realized that the key to eating fewer calories and staying on that diet depends on the diet and the individual.

This realization led me down a new path of inquiry: How can we use what we now know about weight loss to come up with a way to help a dieter determine which diet will work most effectively for her (or him)? More specifically: What list of questions would let you figure out which diet might work best for you? The search for that questionnaire was the genesis of this book.

For the past few years, I've been working to distill my research findings and extrapolate my clinical experience in treating overweight patients into a comprehensive questionnaire that anyone could complete.

Once you've scored your self-test, you'll be able to choose a basic weight-loss diet that best fits you. Using the questionnaire, you will then customize that diet based on specific aspects of how you eat, how you live, and how your body works. The Perfect Fit Questionnaire takes an hour or so to complete, but the results will save *years* of searching for the right diet.

The Perfect Fit Questionnaire will:

- Identify which of the three basic types of diets will work best for you.

- Customize that diet to your medical, personal, and family history, as well as your food preferences, creating an individualized diet that will appeal to your tastebuds and help you lose weight and achieve optimal fitness and health.

- Prescribe a diet and lifestyle plan that you can live with, happily, for the rest of your life.

The Perfect Fit Questionnaire is a direct translation of the doctor-patient Q&A I've been using to design personalized weight-loss plans for my patients. The answers to this questionnaire will empower aspiring dieters—whether obese or merely overweight—to lose weight successfully and keep it off, despite previous failed attempts.

## WHY TASTE MATTERS

The Perfect Fit Diet is based on the idea that a successful diet is one that is built around your life and your preferences. In recent research, food preference has emerged as a key factor in satisfying hunger, and thus in dieting success. (Nutritionists who work with people with diabetes have led the way in recognizing the importance of structuring a diet that works with a dieter's individual tastes.)

The Perfect Fit Questionnaire systematically uncovers what makes you eat, what tastes good to you, what relieves your cravings, and what makes you feel satisfied. It incorporates that information into a personalized diet plan that will let you lose weight and maintain your ideal weight because it's a satisfying eating plan that's a perfect fit for your lifestyle, your food preferences, and your satisfaction—in short, a perfect fit for you.

Doctors, and just about everyone else, have thought of food preference as something trained and therefore malleable. If you want to lose weight, you should learn to love broccoli. If you can't, then you aren't serious about weight loss. Science is beginning to show us how little of food preference is really learned behavior and how much is in our genes. Recent research here at Yale reveals that what we think of as food preference or taste is actually a complex variety of factors, both genetic and acquired, physical and emotional. One of the most interesting findings is that some foods taste very different from one person to another, and that this difference in sensation is genetic. For example, some people have taste buds that are keenly sensitive to even a trace of bitterness, and to them vegetables like broccoli and Brussels sprouts and fruits like grapefruit can be extremely unpalatable.

In experiments, researchers have used a chemical called 6-n-propylthiouracil, or PROP for short, to test for this trait. Some people can detect even a trace of this chemical, while others cannot taste it at all. And it runs in families. If one of your parents has the ability to taste PROP, there's a good chance that you can too.

Researchers at the National Institutes of Health recently identified a gene called TAS2R on chromosome 7. There are five forms of this gene, and which one you inherit determines whether you can even detect this bitter taste or to what degree you are sensitive to it. If you inherit a high degree of sensitivity to bitterness from both parents, you will be able to taste even the tiniest amount of PROP. And if you can taste PROP, then you may not be able to enjoy broccoli, because the bitter flavor of that vegetable will overwhelm its other flavors. This means that hating vegetables may not be so much a moral failing as it is a genetic trait, like hair color or the presence of freckles.

That's just one reason why accommodating individual food preferences is so important to a successful diet. You can't stick with a diet that feeds you foods you hate. Not when there are so many choices out there, right at arm's length, that you love. Deprivation diets only work in the short run; you can only stay on a diet that satisfies your fundamental food cravings. Unless your diet reflects your individual food preferences, it can't be sustained—because it won't be satisfying. The Perfect Fit Diet is the first weight-loss program that respects this immutable law of human nature.

The bottom line of the new science of dieting is clear: If you can customize a diet to reflect your individual profile—your genes, your metabolism, your lifestyle, and your food preferences— you can stay satisfied and stay on your diet. That's how you lose weight.

# CHAPTER 2

# WHY ONE SIZE DOESN'T FIT ALL

THE IDEA THAT ONE size can't fit all should come as no surprise to doctors. We already know it's true when it comes to treating disease. Over the past twenty years, science has made dramatic discoveries in the areas of genetics and physiology, in the way even the smallest cells in the body interact with different medications and other therapies. Using this ever-expanding knowledge base, doctors hope to some day to be able to devise an individualized treatment regimen based on a patient's medical profile, family history, and genetics to control chronic diseases. Take high blood pressure. For the past twenty years, doctors have enjoyed the ability to prescribe one of many drugs that are extremely effective in lowering blood pressure.

It's only been in the last decade, though, that studies have confirmed what doctors already knew in their gut: These medicines have different effects on different people.

In 1993, *The New England Journal of Medicine* published a study by researcher Barry Materson, who compared the effects of six classes of high blood pressure medicines on a group of two thousand veterans. Half of those vets were white; half were African-American. The study showed that African-Americans responded better than whites to a class of antihypertensive drugs known as calcium channel blockers and not as well as whites to another class of medicines known as ACE inhibitors. Why that should be the case is still being investigated. That it is true has been accepted and shapes medical decision making thousands of times a day.

More recently, science has witnessed the birth of an entire field, known as pharmacogenetics, dedicated to the investigation of the inherited mechanisms that determine how we respond to medications. This discipline grew from the widespread recognition that different patients respond differently to the same medications. For example, it has long been known that while codeine is a wonderful pain reliever for most of us, for about 6 percent of the population it offers no relief and no benefit. Why? Because in order to work as a painkiller, codeine has to be broken down into its morphine base. Six to 7 percent of the population is born without the machinery to perform this chemical transformation. This tiny genetic difference has no other effect except to make a good painkiller ineffective.

Here's another example, perhaps a little closer to home. Researchers in Canada wanted to see if obesity had a genetic component in addition to the environmental aspect, which is already well-recognized. They found a group of twins and for several weeks fed them 1,000 calories more than they normally ate. Each twin in the pair gained about the same amount of weight as their siblings. This makes sense, since we all know that the two people who make up any pair of identical twins share the exact same genes. But here's where it got interesting: Different twin sets gained very different amounts of weight—ranging from 10 to 40 pounds—proving that your genes strongly influence how you gain weight. Same "therapy"—overeating by 1,000 calories a day—led to very different results.

The same is turning out to be true for the treatment of obesity. A few years ago, there was a study to see how genes affect weight loss. Again, researchers turned to identical twins, recruiting a couple dozen identical female twins and putting all of them on a reduced-calorie diet. Each set of twins ate a diet that slashed their calorie intake by 1,000 calories. Again, each of the twins in any one pair lost about the same amount of weight but there were big differences in how much weight different sets of twin lost. Same therapy, different results.

## THE SAME, ONLY DIFFERENT

So why should there be differences in how we lose weight? Haven't we all learned that a calorie is a calorie? It's what we've been taught, but we are just beginning to find out that it isn't necessarily so.

For example, there is a segment of the population that processes carbohydrates differently than most of the rest of us. These people are born with a tendency to become resistant to the effects of insulin. They have what we now call metabolic syndrome (more about this later). Because of that difference, when they eat a diet low in fat and high in carbohydrates—the typical weight-loss diet, recommended by most physicians and dieticians—they don't lose weight. In fact they are more likely to gain weight. Why? It turns out that when these folks eat a diet high in carbohydrates, their bodies respond by putting out high levels of insulin. Now, insulin serves a critical purpose in the body—it helps cells take up the sugar made from the carbs. Without it you will certainly die. But because these folks are resistant to insulin, it takes a lot more insulin to get the job done.

High levels of insulin put the body in a fat-storage mode rather than a fat-burning mode, so it's much harder for them to lose weight and many will gain weight on a diet that puts them into a high-insulin state.

And that's not the only difference between these insulin-resistant people and everyone else. When they eat a typical low-fat diet—the kind of diet doctors recommend to lower cholesterol—they develop high cholesterol instead. Thus, the most popular diet among physicians and dietitians today is not the healthiest diet for those with this abnormality known as metabolic syndrome. And it's very common: Twenty percent of the U.S. population has this syndrome. Again, the same therapy will cause a very different effect in some of us.

It is likely that there are other differences between people and the way they process certain foods. For instance, there is good evidence that tiny differences in our fat-processing genes can make dramatic differences in the ways we respond to the amount and type of fat in our diets. That's why on the exact same typical American diet some folks will have normal cholesterol, while others will need medicines to keep their cholesterol down. These mechanisms are still not well understood but are the target of much investigation right now.

## JUST PUSH BACK FROM THE TABLE . . .

There are many differences in the way we process food, and there are just as many differences in the signals that tell us to stop eating. What makes us put down the fork and stop is actually a very complicated little drama and is probably controlled in many ways. However, it seems clear that when it comes to feeling that we've "had enough," different people respond to different cues.

For example, we humans (as well as other species) have what is called sensory-specific satiety. What that means is that the enjoyment of any given flavor or texture begins to decrease as more of that food is eaten. But as that happens, the appetite for other flavors or textures remains unsatisfied. This is why we can feel full after a big meal of meat and potatoes and still find room for dessert. The appetite for sweets was untouched by the meal, and while you may or may not crave them, the sight or thought of them will appeal to your mouth even if your stomach is "full." This is thought to be part of the biological drive that encourages us to eat a variety of foods.

Genetically speaking, this trait comes in handy on the savannahs of Africa if you're an *Australopithecus* primate trying to evolve into a human being. If you're plopped down in front of the TV in the den, this trait has a whole other effect.

This form of feeling satisfied actually takes place in the mouth. We know this because researchers have done experiments where a food was eaten but wasn't allowed to reach the stomach. Research subjects were instructed to treat test foods the way an oenophile might treat wines at a tasting. They were to put the food in their mouths, savor it, then spit it out. Soon enough, they reported feeling they'd had enough of that flavor, even though they actually hadn't eaten any. So one mechanism of fullness derives from having a good variety both in each meal and throughout the entire day. Those who respond strongly to variety may be able to eat a small quantity of a wide variety of foods and feel satisfied. Recent research shows that this is particularly powerful in foods that have strong flavors. This means that for those who respond best to this type of signal, bland "comfort" foods may not be very filling. They can eat and eat and eat but never really feel full because it's not triggering that sense of fullness they get from more flavorful foods.

Other research shows that volume of food is an important cue of satiety. In one experiment, twenty young men were given four different drinks before four meals. The drinks had the same total number of calories but had different amounts of fluid. The young men drank this before eating lunch, and then the amount that each of the men ate at lunch was carefully monitored. The more fluid the men drank, the less they ate at lunch, even though the number of calories in the drinks was the same. So volume of food is an important factor for many people.

A third powerful satiety cue for many people is the richness of a food—that is, how much fat and protein it contains. These foods trigger the release of specific digestive enzymes that not only work to break down these foods but also travel to the brain to report that you have eaten them.

It seems clear that people have different responses to these various satiety cues. What makes us feel full is hardwired into the brain, and like so much of this wiring, it differs from individual to individual. Two studies recently published in *The New England Journal of Medicine* identified a genetic variant that, in a small percentage of obese children, made them produce less of a brain hormone known to cause a feeling of fullness. The clear implication is that these children may have become obese simply because they have never really felt full or satisfied by a meal.

There is also evidence that cues to stop eating can be overwhelmed by other feelings and sensations. This is especially true in those who are overweight and those who diet frequently. So it may well be that once you start gaining weight, it becomes easier to gain more because the body's usual mechanisms for controlling diet are misfiring.

Obviously, if you are trying to reduce the amount of food you eat, then choosing foods that will provide you with the loudest and clearest cues that you've had enough will be an important way to start any good diet. Eating foods that don't relay this key signal to the brain—regardless of how good they may be for you—is going to be frustrating and undermine your willpower.

When you are selecting a diet, you will want one that gives you every possible advantage in staying on it—one that allows you to eat the foods you like and avoid the foods you don't like; one that takes advantage of whichever form of satiety speaks to your body best; one that is best for your body and your health. Can we predict who can stay on a diet and who can't? Anyone who has tried to diet knows that it's not about motivation. The key to being able to stay on a diet is how well that diet fits you as an individual.

*The Perfect Fit for Robert (lost 35 pounds)*
*I'd noticed my weight was really creeping up over the past few years. You know, you get married and suddenly you're eating well; you get involved in your work and end up working more and playing less and suddenly the pounds just start packing on. I noticed, but I didn't really know what to do. I'm not a joiner so all those programs that make you join up didn't appeal to me. And I couldn't believe that those prepackaged meals were going to offer me a long-term solution. I found this book and it appealed to my inner science nerd. I became my own little science project.*

*I knew I had a lot to learn about how I should eat. Viewing myself as a project let me get the kind of distance to really take a look at what I did and what it was doing to me. Doing the questionnaire, I realized I'm a guy who needs a lot of variety in what I eat. Now, that might not always have been true. I know I've made my way through those big 24-oz porterhouse steaks in my time, but at this point in my life I really need to hit the taste buds—that's what's most important to me now. If I get the variety I need, I can do with a lot less of whatever I'm eating. That was the trick—trying to reconcile what my taste buds wanted and what my body wanted. But I think I've mostly figured that out.*

*I don't deprive myself. I really eat whatever I want—if I really want it. But I don't eat all of it, that's for sure. I know that the last bite doesn't taste as good as the first bite and when you know that, it's easier to stop.*

*I eat more regularly now. I noticed that when you eat smaller meals, you get hungry, and then, when it's time to eat, it's time to eat. You have an hour or 2, but you can't go 4–5 hours. And I'm definitely staying away from the ravenous holy-smoke-I-could-eat-a-horse kind of appetite. Because I know, once I'm there, I won't be able to stop eating until I literally can't put another forkful in.*

*I'm not quite at my goal yet, but I'm back into a set of clothes I haven't worn in I don't know how long. I'm down 35 pounds so far. I'd like to lose another 10 and I'm pretty sure I'll get there.*

*I feel better now. I've got more energy; I feel a lot healthier. I needed some direction, but now that I've got it, I'm never going back.*

## YOU'RE ON YOUR OWN

Think about that feeling you have in the supermarket. You are pushing your cart down the aisle. Products scream out to you from the shelf, by color, by name, by packaging—they shout, "Buy me!" And it's hard to resist. The choices are intentionally overwhelming. The possibilities of what you could eat are almost endless. And who is in the supermarket making these decisions? Often, just you. All by yourself.

This, it should be said, is pretty new. For most of the history of the species, there was something else accompanying any person who was trying to make the decision about what to eat. It was called culture. If you were Italian, or even Italian-American, there was this whole tradition of eating called Italian food. The same was true regardless of where you came from: Culture defined diet. There were cuisines—Sephardic Jewish, Irish, Hopi, Hawaiian, German-American. Cultural menus were largely inherited. And what were they? They were the passed-down wisdom of a people about what was good, healthy, and available to eat in a particular place. This was what culture did. It set the framework for people's diets.

Today, your cultural tradition is no match for the supermarket, where, increasingly, one is able to assemble the essentials of every world cuisine. Market forces have overwhelmed culture. What that means is that we must all create our own private cuisine—an individual culture that's just about you and all the choices that are out there.

The power of supermarket choices cannot be overemphasized.

One of the forgotten stories about the fall of communism locates the precise moment when the wall started to crumble: It was in a Western supermarket. The story is told by Vasily Aksyonov, a Russian writer who had fled his homeland. He recalled a time in the late 1970s when the Soviet Minister of Agriculture was visiting Canada. The hosting officials took the Soviet bureaucrat to a supermarket. He walked up and down the aisles in stunned disbelief. How could this be? How could anyone have this much choice, this much food just sitting on a shelf waiting to be bought? He noticed the aisles filled with people leisurely walking about, plucking one thing or another from the shelves, and came to the conclusion that the entire store was a setup. He was convinced that the supermarket was a "Potemkin village," a fake set filled with all these goods and tricked out with actors playing the roles of customers. And why? Just to make the Soviet visitor feel bad. He thought about life back home and how the average family bartered and bargained to get a simple staple like a tomato or a turnip. This display was just absurd in its excess. Really, he concluded, the Westerners had practically made fools of themselves with this obviously phony store.

After the tour, the minister got back into his limo and headed toward another meeting with officials. On the way, they happened to pass another supermarket. The minister ordered the car to stop. Smiling slyly, he said he would like to visit a supermarket not officially scheduled for the tour. So they parked, and apparently the first crack sending a fissure up the wall of communism occurred when that minister—a man named Mikhail Gorbachev—stepped through the automatic doors and saw the same scene he'd observed at the last store—the unreal amount of choice, the customers wandering the aisles.

It's hard for us to imagine just how peculiar supermarkets are in the history of humankind. They were invented after World War II and represented a sharp turn in the history of eating. For the first time in the history of food, each of us can choose to eat just about anything. The market has done what it does at its best—provide choice. Now we are swimming in it, and there is nothing between each one of us and the mountain of food out there except the way we as individuals decide to eat.

*The Perfect Fit for Lillian (lost 20 pounds)*

*Diet, exercise, and weight did not enter my consciousness until I gave birth to my second child in 20 months. I was 29 and had the two babies so close together that I never had the opportunity to lose the weight from the first child before I got pregnant with the second one. Plus, I was in my first year of practicing law and so I had very little time to even think about exercising. All I knew was that I felt fat and that it did not feel good. My solution at the time was to eat almost nothing but rice cakes for about 6 months. The pounds came off but I hated every minute of it.*

*After I lost the weight, I joined an aerobics class and with the exercise I found I could eat pretty much whatever I wanted and not gain weight.*

*Then, I turned 40, and I noticed that the exercise-every-day-and-eat-whatever-I-wanted approach wasn't working any more. I was gaining a few pounds every year. My doctor noticed and she wasn't concerned, but I was. My clothes didn't fit any more, my size was moving upward, and I was starting to look matronly. It was hard to look at myself in the mirror.*

*I knew I couldn't do the rice cakes again. It was tough then—it would be impossible now. There had to be a better way than just starving myself. I started cruising the aisles of the diet-book section of my local bookstore, picking up diet books I'd heard of and quite a few I hadn't. That's when I turned to* The Perfect Fit Diet. *It just made sense.*

*So I took it home to give it a shot. Keeping the diary, filling out the questionnaire was a real education. It forced me to think about what I was putting in my mouth. And why. I realized they were both important. By analyzing what and how I really ate and identifying the foods that I really liked I was able to change the way I ate. Not dramatically, just rationally. I came to understand what was good about the way I ate and what was causing me to gain weight. I started to pay attention not just to what I ate, but how much I ate. I figured out which of the foods I was eating carried the most satisfaction.*

*I eat a pretty low-fat diet, and so I wasn't surprised when the questionnaire directed me to the Counting Fats Diet. I didn't realize that my job was making me fat by keeping me too busy to snack when I got hungry between meals. Using the meal plans as a template, I added a little more protein to the meals I ate and made sure I had a little something to nosh if that didn't hold me. As crazy as my days can get, I found that if I had a little package of peanuts or a cheese stick I could make it to dinner hungry, but not starving. With a few tweaks to my diet, the 20 pounds that I wanted to lose seemed to slide off. I "dieted" with remarkably little effort, without feeling deprived.*

*Knowledge is power and now I know. And because I know, I'm certain that I'll never have to fight those extra 20 pounds again.*

## "I'M GOING ON A DIET!"

People say things like, "Hey, I'm on a diet," or "I'm going on a diet." Doctors don't talk this way (or they shouldn't) because they know that we're all on a diet—a diet is simply what you eat. And that diet either works for you—lets you feel good and maintain a weight that also feels good—or it doesn't.

There are two aspects of traditional weight-loss dieting that bear commenting on. First, when you diet, you actually think about what you are going to eat and try to take control of that activity. This is the positive aspect of dieting.

Let's compare that to what happens under normal circumstances, when habit and the vast commercial forces determine what you eat. Most of us eat out of the home at least one meal a day—often even more—and if you don't brown-bag it, the food choices we have to make are limited by what's available where we are when we need to eat. William Shakespeare said, "There's small choice in rotten apples," yet that's the type of choice we have far too often when we have to eat away from home.

We know that, and so when we are dieting we know to plan ahead so that we don't have to either eat what's there or not eat at all. Planning what we eat is something we should do all the time, even when we're not trying to lose weight.

Here's the downside of dieting: We think of it as a temporary aberration, a deviation from our normal way of eating. This second assumption is what leads to so much of what is wrong with the whole culture of dieting.

First of all, if we accept the idea that a diet is temporary, then any diet can be tolerated if it isn't for long. That's why it doesn't matter if the foods on the diet are the foods you like to eat—it's just temporary, until you lose the weight—and then you can go back to the old ways once again. In fact, in some ways it's *better* if you don't like the foods. If you don't like them—goes this argument—you won't eat as much and you will lose the weight even faster. But that's a fallacy; you won't be able to eat foods you hate—at least not for long.

Second, if you think of a diet as temporary and different from the way you normally eat, a weight-loss diet allows you to avoid thinking about some of the ways that your *real* diet contributes to your difficulties in managing your weight. A weight-loss diet cannot teach you anything about the way you normally eat. A rotation diet or one that emphasizes only one food, which causes weight loss by severely restricting choice, has nothing to offer in a world where choices are practically limitless. It's just not realistic.

Albert Einstein once defined insanity as asking the same question over and over and each time expecting a different answer. If that is true, we are a nation of nuts. We go on weight-loss diets to get rid of the weight our "real" diets have put on us. Then, whether we are successful in our weight-loss diet or not, we go back to our old diet and, whad'ya know, if it made us gain weight before, it will do it again, because nothing has happened to change that diet.

In order to change what your diet does, you have to change your diet. If you just have a fling with some new and different weight-loss program, you may or may not lose weight, but you probably won't stay on that program forever. *You have to change the way you eat every day.* And that is not easy. (I don't have to tell you that. If you are reading this book, you are probably all too familiar with the difficulty of changing basic behavior.)

So, how can we change such fundamental behavior? I would argue that you have to work with what you have and try to shape that basic template into a diet that will work for you.

Over these next chapters, I will walk you through the techniques that will help you design *your* perfect diet. You will learn to identify the foods you love and can't live without. Then you will learn how to put them together to create a diet that is both satisfying and good for you. You will learn what your eating triggers are and how to avoid them. You will learn how you respond to stress and how to keep that from ruining an otherwise perfect diet. Finally, you will figure out how to increase the activity level in your life to reduce stress and help you achieve and maintain your ideal weight.

I can't promise you it will be easy, but you already know that changing the way you eat is a tall order. What I can promise is that it is possible to create a diet that works and that still allows you to enjoy what you eat and eat what you love. In fact, that's the only way to lose weight and keep it off.

# CHAPTER 3

# HOW THE PERFECT FIT DIET WORKS

THERE ARE LOTS OF different weight-loss diets out there that work for different people. So how do you span the distance between you and your Perfect Fit Diet?

It's a customizing process that I sometimes compare to tailoring a suit. First, you find the basic pattern that fits your style; then you tailor the suit to your particular figure; finally, you accessorize to make it a perfect fit for your personal tastes and lifestyle.

Over the course of this book, I'm going to walk you through the steps you need to take to create your Perfect Fit Diet:

- Step 1: Keep a 4-day eating and exercise diary.*

- Step 2: Fill out the Perfect Fit Questionnaire.

- Step 3: Score the questionnaire to identify which of the three basic diet types is right for you—the Counting Carbohydrates Diet, the Counting Calories Diet, or the Counting Fats Diet.

- Step 4: Customize that diet based on your food preferences and family medical history.

- Step 5: Customize your diet to fit your lifestyle—exercise, eating patterns, family and work life—to create an eating and exercise plan that fits your long-term weight goals.

## Step 1: The Eating and Exercise Diary

First, you will need to keep an eating diary for 4 days, writing down everything you eat and drink over the course of those days. Try to include 2 workdays and then the weekend. Studies show that we eat differently (and often more) on the weekends when compared to the weekdays. From a doctor's perspective, the diary is the equivalent to taking a detailed patient history. You need to know precisely how, what, and why you eat. The eating diary is the most important part of the information that you'll need to collect in order to fill out the Perfect Fit Questionnaire correctly.

During the days that you are keeping the eating diary, you may find yourself wondering, "Should I put that in the diary?" The answer will always be "yes." No matter what it is, if it went into your mouth and you swallowed it, write it down.

This goes for drinks as well. Even water. Write everything down. Everything. Trust me, the difference between what you think you eat

*A number of readers told me that they simply couldn't wait the 4 days to start the diet. They just didn't have the patience. I think the diary is important, but I recognize that some of you will want to skip this step, so I have developed the Jump-Start version of the questionnaire, which allows you to fill it out and score it without a diary.

and what you actually eat and write down is so dramatic that I have yet to have a patient return with a diary who wasn't simply flabbergasted by what he found himself reading after those few days. Here's what a number of studies have discovered: You won't remember eating it or drinking it if you don't write it down. So write it down.

Meanwhile, I want you to keep a parallel diary of your exercise and other physical activities. As with food, we tend to avoid looking at our level of physical activity—or inactivity. Your exercise diary will give you a good overview of what level of physical activity you gravitate toward, what you enjoy, and what you avoid.

## Step 2: The Perfect Fit Questionnaire—To Diet Successfully, Know Thyself

The true secret to successful weight loss is "know thyself." Know what you need, both physically and psychologically, from food and how to satisfy those needs in a way that's compatible with weight loss. Self-knowledge around our food needs is more complicated than it sounds. Perhaps nowhere do physical and emotional issues connect more deeply than in our relationship with food.

The Perfect Fit Questionnaire is an in-depth exercise in self-discovery. It is a series of eighty-three questions about what, when, why, and how you eat. It draws upon what you know you like and what you know makes you feel full. The questionnaire systematically uncovers the obvious and not-so-obvious truths about your individual medical history, family history, and food and weight history. It investigates the exercise and stress levels in your life. In addition to your own medical history, it asks about your parents' and siblings' medical history. Using that basic data, the questionnaire can help you identify patterns of how you gain weight and how you can lose it.

The quiz is broken into fifteen sections of one to nine questions each. Each of these sections identifies some meaningful aspect of the relationship between you and that complex calculus of intake (food) and output (activity) that describes you at your current weight. The first two sections focus on food preferences. (The Jump-Start version of the questionnaire also identifies aspects of your food preferences using questions that don't require a 4-day diary to answer.) The questions show you if you are a "Carnimore," someone who can't imagine life without meat; a "Milk Mavin," who needs the cheese with the crackers; a sweets lover; or a "Junk-Food Junkie." All these preferences shape your current diet and will shape your perfect diet as well.

Then we try to figure out what makes you full. Some of my patients tell me that they can't feel full unless they eat a certain amount of food. They just aren't satisfied eating less, no matter how many calories they take in. Still others feel cravings for specific tastes or textures. They find themselves standing in front of the refrigerator scanning the shelves for . . . something. Maybe it's a crunch; maybe it's a taste of something sweet; maybe it's something sour or hot. If they can figure out what they are hungering for, they can eat a bit of that and finally be satisfied. If not, they find themselves eating other things and, too often, still not getting that satisfied feeling. All of us have multiple ways of feeling full; figure out which ones are important for you, and you will be able to feel full and eat less by specifically directing your eating to answer that hunger.

The questionnaire also asks about your medical history. If you are healthy and under 25, then your own history may not be as important as the history of your parents or siblings. Diet and activity have a tremendous impact on your likelihood of developing many diseases that have a hereditary component to them. For example, diabetes is much more common in those with a family history of diabetes. If you are overweight or inactive, your risk is even greater. Hypertension, too, is far more common in those with a family history of high blood pressure. So medical history, both yours and your family's, will also figure into the diet that works best for you.

Eating habits are key in dieting. Do you skip breakfast? Do you eat only one meal a day? Do you snack? Do you need to nibble? Do you eat regular meals, or is your life too hectic to allow the traditional three squares? Do you eat out often? Which meals? Who cooks in your household? Who shops? All of these issues will have an impact on your Perfect Fit Diet.

What about emotional eating? Are you a stress eater? Do you eat when you're bored? When you're angry? When you need a reward? Understanding your eating triggers is an essential part of constructing a diet that works for you.

Finally, let's look at your level of activity. Do you always take the elevator? Do you always drive to the store? Are there ways to increase the amount of daily activity in your life? And what about exercise? Do you walk? Do you run? Do you swim? Have you ever exercised? Why did you stop? What keeps you from exercising now? Being active is essential to weight loss and to weight-loss maintenance. Our job is to help you find an activity—or even better, several activities—that will fit comfortably into your life.

Once you collect all this data, you're ready to score the questionnaire and find out which diet fits you best.

## Step 3: Identify Which Basic Diet Is Right for You

Diets that help you lose weight do so by reducing the number of calories you take in and increasing the amount of energy you use up. Having said that, different diets use different strategies to achieve those ends.

Most diets reduce your calorie intake by restricting access to one or more types of foods. Once you recognize this, it's easy to classify the vast panoply of diets onto a sort of spectrum based on what exactly they are limiting.

At one end are the very low-fat (high-carbohydrate) diets offered by Dean Ornish, M.D., and Neal Bernard, M.D. Both recommend extraordinary reductions in fat intake. Dr. Ornish recommends a

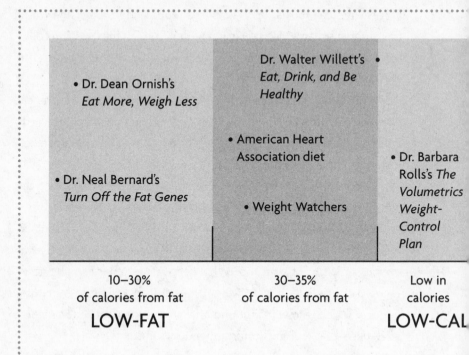

vegetarian diet; Dr. Bernard goes even further to recommend a vegan diet in which you eat no animal products whatsoever. A little further up the spectrum you get the more moderate fat restrictions where you're allowed to eat some fat, but only the so-called good fat. These would include diets recommended by the American Heart Association and Weight Watchers, and the Harvard diet as designed by Walter Willett, M.D., Dr.P.H. These generally recommend that you restrict your fat intake to 30 to 35 percent of the calories you eat.

Right smack in the middle, you get diets that focus on cutting calories. These diets come in two basic flavors. There are those that offer unlimited amounts of a few low-calorie foods. Rotation diets—like the recent cabbage soup diet—use this strategy. More commonly, calorie-counting diets focus on portion control and offer a much wider variety of foods, emphasizing foods that provide a greater sense of fullness and satisfaction with fewer calories. Usually, they promote

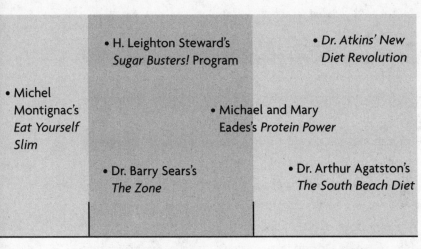

• H. Leighton Steward's
*Sugar Busters!* Program

• Dr. Atkins' New
*Diet Revolution*

• Michel
Montignac's
*Eat Yourself
Slim*

• Michael and Mary
Eades's *Protein Power*

• Dr. Barry Sears's
*The Zone*

• Dr. Arthur Agatston's
*The South Beach Diet*

40–20%
of calories from carbs

Less than 20%
of calories from carbs

**LOW-CARB**

foods that are high in fiber, low on the glycemic index, or both. For example, Volumetrics is a calorie-counting diet, although author Barbara Rolls, Ph.D., a researcher at Pennsylvania State University, talks about it in terms of calorie per volume of food or calorie density. On this diet, you can eat more low-density foods than high-density foods.

As we move further up the spectrum, we start seeing diets that focus on limiting carbohydrates. The Zone diet says that you should restrict your carbohydrate intake to just 40 percent of the calories you eat in the course of a day. Around there is the Sugar Busters diet, too, which makes refined carbohydrates and sugars completely off-limits; Protein Power is another diet that limits access to carbs but wants you to replace those carbs with protein rather than fats. And finally, at the outermost edge of the spectrum, are Dr. Atkins' Diet Revolution and the South Beach diet, which seek to reduce your carb intake to the lowest you can tolerate.

Let's take a closer look at these many different diets. While the range might suggest that the choice of diet is arbitrary, I believe that there are particular dieters who do best on each of these diets.

**So who would do well on a diet that primarily restricts fat?** Let's start with food preference. Those who don't eat a lot of meat to begin with would do better than big-time Carnimores. You have to enjoy fruits and vegetables, and having a good appreciation for whole-grain foods would help. Furthermore, this diet is best for people who need volume to feel full. In terms of health, I would recommend this as one possible diet for those with high cholesterol but would not recommend such a diet for those who have diabetes or who process carbohydrates abnormally. (I'll explain how to determine if you fit in this group later, as you score the questionnaire.)

When you eat a high-carb, low-fat diet, eating regular meals is particularly important since there is less fat and protein to make your feeling of fullness last. Finally, a low-fat diet is very hard to keep up with if you travel a lot and eat out frequently. Fresh fruits and veggies and whole-grain foods will make up most of what you eat, and very little of that food is available away from home.

**What about a calorie-counting diet?** This is for folks who need a lot of variety in their diets and for whom portion size is a manageable issue. If you can't eat a little of something you like, a low-calorie diet may not be for you. On the other hand, if you find yourself standing in front of the refrigerator, trying to identify the food you are craving, you may do very well on a diet that allows you to eat some of whatever you crave and that purposefully offers a variety of flavors and textures every day.

**Finally, how about a carbohydrate-counting diet?** This is a diet for eaters who enjoy meat, cheese, and eggs and find it hard to feel full without them. It helps if you don't care much about variety because you often end up eating the same food every day. You have to be able to live in a world with limited fruits and vegetables. And, of course, you have to say good-bye to breads, pastas, and sweets. It is a very restrictive diet, and yet there are many who have successfully lost weight on this diet and can maintain their weight using these principles. Portion control is an important aspect of this diet, too, although it may be less of an issue because of the filling quality of proteins and fats. People who travel or eat out a lot often do well on this type of diet, because easily found entrées of grilled meat, chicken, or fish plus a salad make up the prototypical meal of this diet.

After you figure out which diet plan is right for you, I'll instruct you to turn to the section about that diet in part 3. There, I give a brief summary of the principles of each diet. Following that is a list of foods that work with that diet and a 7-day eating plan to help you implement the diet in your own home. I have developed a version of each diet based on my own research. In general, the meal plans I recommend are rich in fresh fruits and vegetables and feature foods that are low in saturated fats and that have a low glycemic load. Following the diet and food recommendations in your Perfect Fit Diet plan, you will have the fundamentals of the low-fat, low-calorie, or low-carbohydrate diet that will work for you.

## Step 4: Customize Your Basic Diet to Your Food Preferences and Medical History

Once you figure out which diet is best for you, you can shape it even further based on how you answer the individual sections of the questionnaire. Each section is designed to help you define a specific aspect of the way you eat. Once you have defined the various aspects of your diet, I will try to help you tailor your diet around this aspect that is uniquely you.

**Food preferences.** Food preference plays a role in customizing your diet. All classes of foods have some good in them. Our job is to look at the kinds of foods you like and understand what's good in these foods and what's not so good. Using that knowledge, you can customize your diet to maximize the healthy qualities of the foods you love while minimizing those qualities that are less healthy.

In a diet that tries, as this one does, to outsmart the forces that help us put on weight and make it hard to lose it, there can be no forbidden foods. All is allowed, but you have to plan for it. I think what too many people do is simply decide to say no to a food that they love but believe has contributed to their inability to control their weight. They decide that this food—say, a treat that is sweet or salty, filled with sugar or fat or both—may never be eaten again.

Two things happen when you do that: First, when you eat the thing that you love, it will be unplanned—you won't have any room left in your diet for it. And that's what usually happens. When you forbid yourself to have something, you end up eating it on top of everything else you eat. That doesn't work. Since you are going to have it, you need to count it, and the only way to do that is to plan for it.

Something else happens when you know that a food is off-limits: That knowledge often drives you to eat too much of it, since you feel that you will never be able to eat it again. This is one of the ways that dieting changes your relationship to food, and one that can be avoided. If you are going to incorporate a new way of eating into your life, which I hope is your goal, you have to figure out some way to make peace with the foods you love and how to fit them into a diet that's perfect for you. This is one of the goals of customizing your diet.

**Medical history.** Your medical and family history must play a role in customizing your diet. For example, if you have a family history of high cholesterol, chances are you will not end up on a carbohydrate-counting diet. In addition, there are ways to shape your diet so that the fats you eat will help you bring down rather than ratchet up your cholesterol.

## Step 5: Customize Your Basic Diet to Fit Your Lifestyle

What you eat, how you eat, and when you eat—these are all essential characteristics of your lifestyle. And despite what we nutrition buffs would like to think, chances are they are not the most important issues of your life. Instead, they must compete with other compelling aspects of your day: your job, your family, and all the other pleasures and obligations that make up a life. But the life into which you integrate this diet will have a profound effect on how it works. Therefore, you need to take your real life into consideration when you design your diet.

Usually, when a diet gets out of hand and causes weight gain, it is due not only to the foods eaten but also to when, where, why, and how the food is eaten. As adults, overcommitted, wildly busy, terrifically stressed, we have developed eating habits that interfere with natural mechanisms that regulate when and how much we eat. Normally, we eat a variety of foods but take in more or less the same number of calories each day. We haven't figured out how we can do this—but we can. And thanks to this very finely tuned system, we are usually able to regulate our intake without even thinking about it so that it doesn't vary more than 100 calories or so day in and day out.

But far too often how we eat undermines this built-in regulator. Stressed-out and busy workers or parents can find themselves too busy to eat. Maybe we grab a quick snack, or maybe we just tough it out, but in either case chances are that when our next meal rolls around we are starving. We sit down and in an instant consume our entire meal and more—often much more. The mechanisms that might otherwise tell us that we have eaten enough are silenced by our outsize hunger and we overeat. Happens all the time.

And then there is the opposite problem: Some of us eat when we aren't hungry. Maybe we are stressed, bored, or tired, but we're not hungry.

The problem is that your body treats these snacks differently from the snacks you eat when you're hungry. Snacks that you eat when you're hungry usually cause you to eat less at your next meal than you otherwise would eat. Snacks that you eat when you're not hungry don't do that. Your body just doesn't count them when it's doing the math about how many calories you've eaten. So food you eat when you're not hungry is *extra* calories.

If you travel frequently, your food choices are limited by what is available to travelers—and those are often some sad choices. Your diet has to make room for your travel. Even if you are not on the road a lot, you may eat out frequently. Again, this is a challenge when you are trying to control what you eat. Your diet has to make room for eating out—it's as simple as that.

Working long hours often leaves us feeling that there is no time to take care of ourselves. While we can't add to the 24 hours that make up our day, in every life there has to be room to eat and drink and exercise, and while choices may be limited, there are still choices. This book will help you know which choices will work best for you.

I also hope I'm able to persuade you that one of those choices will be to integrate a higher level of activity into your life. You can lose weight without exercising. Many studies support that. But it's much harder to *maintain* weight loss without exercise, and most studies show that too. I know that exercise can seem silly and too difficult to integrate into a busy life, but there is every reason in the world to believe that it is a necessary part of a healthy life. Our job is to figure out a way for you to sneak some exercise into your leisure. To do this, you need to find the activities that suit you and emphasize those. I can't promise you that exercise will help you lose weight, but I can promise that it will make you feel better and that *that* will help you lose weight.

# HOW THE PERFECT FIT DIET WORKS: SHELLEY

So, how does this work in real life? Let's go back to my sister Shelley. She's 48 years old and has been overweight for most of her life. When she found out that I was putting this questionnaire together, she begged me to let her be the first person to try it. So, I assigned her homework—create a food diary and collect her basic medical info—and then we reconvened.

## Steps 1 and 2: The Eating Diary and the Questionnaire

As we went through her food diary, once again I was reminded of how useful and instructive this exercise is. I say this even though I know my sister very well.

Except for a couple of years just before puberty, we have always been the best of friends. Even though we haven't lived in the same state since high school, we talk almost daily and visit frequently. I bet I know her better than anyone else on earth. And I'd say she knows me just as well. But I got a whole new education about my sister by going through this diary. Over the years, when we've spoken about diets, she has always raved about the low-carb Scarsdale diet or the Atkins diet. Because of that, I just assumed that she ate a lot of meat and not so many veggies. Wrong.

She did eat meat every day, often at two meals, but she also ate lots of carbs: fruits, pasta, salads, sweets. Going on a low-carb diet, which had worked in the past, was going to be a big change for her. And a big change means probably not sustainable—her history supported this.

When I asked her about these low-carb diets she's had success with in the past, she made an astonishing admission. She told me that one of the reasons that low-carb diets worked for her was because they were so very different from her usual pattern of eating. That difference somehow helped her remember that she was supposed to be losing weight. Also, they prohibited some of the things that she didn't want to moderate, like sweets. And—something else I didn't know about my sister—she thought it was easier to give up sweets for a while than to learn to work with them. So these diets, by prohibiting all carbs, allowed her to avoid the sweets she so often craved—while the diet lasted. But sweets did show up in her food diary. She had a clear weakness for cookies, chocolate, and something called a McFlurry.

Another important clue to which diet she should go on: When asked what she most valued in her diet, she said food variety—it was more important than eating more food and more important than eating rich foods.

## Step 3: Identify Which Basic Diet Plan Is the Right One

When you add all that together—lots of meat at mealtimes, lots of carbs, a passion for sweets, and a need for variety—it becomes clear what kind of diet would suit Shelley best: a diet that counts calories. One that allows her to eat all kinds of foods, just not too much. A 1,200-calorie diet would allow her to lose 1 to 2 pounds per week, and when she approached her target weight, she could increase that slowly to a 1,500-calorie diet to maintain her weight.

## Step 4: Customize the Basic Diet to Food Preferences and Medical History

Food preference was pretty clear: Shelley was a "Carnimore," someone who likes to eat meat daily; she was also a "VegeCarian," big into fresh fruits and vegetables. She loved pasta, so she was a "Starch Stealer." Finally, she was a "Sweets Eater" and needed to make room in her diet for an occasional taste of something sweet. We talked about how to incorporate each of these foods into her diet. She liked variety and was sure to get lots of it; the biggest concern for her was going to be portion control.

You also need to customize for medical history. For Shelley, this was pretty easy. Her BMI was 28—not too bad—and her waist 30 inches. (Women with waists greater than 35 inches are at increased risk for heart disease.) She had no chronic diseases: Her blood pressure ran in the 100/70 range, and her cholesterol was well controlled with a low LDL and high HDL. She's never had any surgery, and she took no medications. She didn't drink or smoke. She lives with her husband and her dog.

Her family history was also good. No history of heart disease, high blood pressure, or diabetes in anyone. These are important questions, since if you have any of these illnesses or risk factors, you have to recognize that you're at increased risk yourself. She doesn't, so at least until menopause, these aren't important issues in her diet.

## Step 5: Customize the Basic Diet to Fit the Lifestyle

My sister runs a small but growing business out of her own home, and she has maybe five full-time employees and anywhere from five to ten part-timers. Like all small-business owners, she finds running her own business exciting and stressful.

Most weekdays, she doesn't have breakfast—just a cup of coffee with fat-free milk. She doesn't snack, so by the time lunch rolls around, she's pretty hungry. Her kitchen is right next to the office, which could be convenient, but she doesn't like to cook when her employees are there, and she feels self-conscious about eating in front of them, too. So most days she goes out for lunch with her husband, who also runs his own business from home.

She doesn't have an afternoon snack and often works late after her employees have gone home. She and her husband usually eat late and eat out for dinner maybe four nights a week.

Snacks are often grabbed on the way out the door or in the car when a meal has been missed. Stress eating usually occurs in the early evening as she's winding up the business of the day and is alone in the office.

Exercise helps with the stress, but when the stress is highest, she complains that she has the least time to exercise. When she does exercise, she either catches an aerobics class at a nearby studio or jogs on a treadmill at home. She likes to exercise at lunchtime but often doesn't have time for it. Based on Shelley's answers about her lifestyle, the Perfect Fit Questionnaire recommended the following:

1. Eat three meals a day with healthy snacks available for between-meal hunger.

2. Try not to ignore your hunger until you are famished. Eat when you are hungry, not when you are starving.

3. While you are working to lose weight, limit your eating out to one or two meals per week.

4. When you do go out to eat, order a juice or light soup as an appetizer, then order only a small appetizer for the entrée. If that won't be enough, order a small salad as well.

5. On the weekends, prepare food ahead that will be easy to warm up on those tired evenings when you just can't cook.

6. Keep track of what you eat every day; tally the calories at the end of each meal. Continue the food diary.

7. Prepare your menu for the week on Sunday and prepare as much of it as you can ahead of time.

8. Have a target number of calories for 2 or 3 days—not just per day—so that you can accommodate good days and bad days.

9. Build variety into your exercise plan. Find an aerobics class that fits your schedule and use that at least 2 or 3 days per week.

10. Exercise at home (on your treadmill) on days when you're too busy to go out to exercise.

So that's how it should work with my sister, and so far, so good. It's been over a year now and she's been able to keep losing, although holidays and other interruptions in her routine have been tough. Her weight is down just over 20 pounds—not at her target, but still moving in the right direction.

## HOW THE PERFECT FIT DIET WORKS: MATT

Matt is a 40-year-old businessman with cropped, dark curls and deep dimples that appear and disappear as he speaks. Although he'd been an athlete in college, marriage and a successful career had cut the time he was able to work out, and he had put the pounds on. The year before we first met, he weighed 283 pounds and his cholesterol was 300. But then his father died suddenly of a massive heart attack, and Matt realized that if he didn't lose weight, he could be next. Over the course of the next year, Matt lost almost 100 pounds by working out every day and obsessively limiting his calories to 800 calories a day. When he got within 20 pounds of his dream weight of 160, he was elated.

But almost immediately, he began to put the weight back on. When he passed 200 pounds, he became frantic, desperate. Every day he would pledge to limit his calories to less than 800 a day; most days he ate three or four times that many. He couldn't bring himself to work out, because he hated to see how he looked in shorts. He even tried to make himself vomit after a binge when he ate the icing off a huge rectangular cake, then threw out the rest of the cake. That's when he knew he needed help. His question was, "How can I stop this yo-yoing and maintain a reasonable weight?"

## Steps 1 and 2: The Eating Diary and Questionnaire

Matt weighed 201 pounds at 5 feet 8 inches for a BMI of 30. He already exercised pretty regularly, lifting weights 3 days a week. He ate a good breakfast of fruit and oatmeal every morning. Lunch at the office was a small salad, dried beans, or dried soup, and he fixed a pretty healthy dinner most nights of the week for himself, his wife, and his two teenage daughters.

What he ate at mealtime was low-fat and high-carbohydrate and in small portions. He usually had chicken or fish. Lots of potatoes. Huge amounts of fruit. Good fiber content. So why was he overweight? It was what he ate between mealtimes. Also, as big-time executive, he found himself going out to lunch three times per week. But beyond that, Matt was a stress eater. Matt's preference was chocolate, and there was plenty of it in his office. When the stress was on, Matt would wander through the office, talking with various people about whatever the problem was and all the time munching chocolate that he seemed to find just about everywhere.

At home, Matt had a different problem: After dinner, he often found himself sitting in front of the TV set eating cookies, crackers, nuts, or whatever he could find.

In terms of health, Matt was doing pretty well. He had high cholesterol but his blood pressure was good. He didn't smoke, drank only occasionally, and exercised regularly. His mom was still alive and in great shape.

## Step 3: Identify Which Basic Diet Plan Is the Right One

Based on what Matt already ate, and since he was a middle-aged man with high cholesterol and fat, which accumulated around his waist (the most dangerous kind of fat), I knew he would do well with a low-fat diet. The questionnaire showed the same. For that he needed to restrict his fat intake to 30–35 percent of his calories with less than 7 percent coming from saturated fats. The only oil he should use is olive oil or other monounsaturated oils like canola, or polyunsaturated oil like corn oil.

## Step 4: Customize the Basic Diet to Food Preferences and Medical History

Matt eats lots of potatoes but avoids the leafy greens we usually recommend. Most likely he's a PROP taster (more on that later) and is avoiding vegetables with even a trace of bitterness in them. I directed him to vegetables that he hadn't listed in his food diary but that he might enjoy if he were a PROP taster. I told him to eat more artichokes, asparagus, avocado, carrots, corn, and squash, and eat more fruits, which he seems to love. He also loves rice and beans, which is very helpful on a low-fat diet. I asked him to consider rice and bean dishes as an entrée at least once a week, to experiment with soy products like tofu, and to try whole-grain pastas.

## Step 5: Customize the Basic Diet to Fit the Lifestyle

Matt eats out a lot and feels compelled to clean his plate, training that starts early and is hard to get over. My advice to him is the same as my advice to Shelley: When you are trying to lose weight, limit eating out to one or two meals per week. And when you do eat out, order a light soup or juice, and then an appetizer or even two. Avoid bread. Avoid alcohol.

More important: Matt lets himself get too hungry between breakfast and supper. It is particularly important on a low-fat diet to eat three meals a day and have healthy snacks available. Don't ignore your hunger until you are starving. Eat when you are hungry.

On days he doesn't go out to lunch, Matt starves himself with small meals. He's proud of the fact that most days he eats less than 500 calories (in meals) before getting home from work. Clearly, he needs more than that. No wonder he runs around his office munching on everyone's chocolate—he's starving. He needs to eat three real meals a day and planned snacks as needed. That way other people's snacks won't be so tempting.

Matt obviously needs a bigger lunch. He also needs one that combines foods. He's eating all carbohydrates for his lunch and clearly that's not cutting it. He needs a lunch that combines carbs with more filling proteins and something sweet, like a piece of fruit. If he gets hungry after lunch, he should eat an afternoon snack before he goes home and starts cooking.

Finally, he needs to stop that late-night noshing in front of the TV set. Matt is not alone—eating and watching TV have probably replaced baseball as the great American pastime. It's no accident; research shows that there is a food-related ad on prime-time TV about every 6 minutes. The majority of those ads are for foods with low nutritional value—better known as junk foods. With this type of constant reminder, no wonder those activities get linked together. If Matt eats more food earlier in the day, the need to nosh will diminish. But the habit of watching and eating will remain unless he forces himself out of it.

On the other hand, Matt's exercise level is pretty good. He lifts weights three times a week. Hard to improve on that. But I recommended that he add another exercise to his repertoire—maybe cycling or running on the days he doesn't lift—to give him more of an aerobic workout. Those who like to exercise should build a variety of exercises into their schedule.

Matt made great progress from the start. On a 33-percent-fat diet and his fabulous exercise habit, he lost about 15 pounds over 4 months. He's happy there, and his weight has remained stable.

So how's he doing it? Lunch is working well. He reports that he has a kitchen at his office, and once a week or so he shops for stuff to keep in the kitchen for lunch. He uses the time he spends making lunch to think stuff over. His biggest crisis came a couple of months ago when he changed jobs. With the new job came new obligations to lunch out and, of course, new stress. He's found a restaurant in the area that serves low-fat food that he likes. And he's found a couple of appetizers that work as a meal for him.

He's also enjoyed the variety in his exercise plan. He now swims a couple of times a week and cycles with his kids on the weekends.

And he's healthier too. His cholesterol is down so much that his doctor took him off his medicine. He feels more energetic, happier, sexier. And since he's the household cook, his wife has lost 15 pounds, and she's feeling good too.

## WHAT THE PERFECT FIT DIET CAN DO FOR YOU

Shelley and Matt are just two of the formerly failed dieters I meet every week in my clinical practice. They see their lapses as proof of their weak wills. But dieting isn't about moral strength—it's about compatibility between diet and dieter, finding a way to eat that you can enjoy and that allows you to include the foods you love while you lose weight. My five-step strategy will lead you to the diet that is perfect for you.

My patients have done it. You can, too.

PART

# THE PERFECT FIT
# QUESTIONNAIRE

# CHAPTER 4
## GETTING STARTED

B EFORE YOU TURN TO the questionnaire, you will have to do a little research. You already know that you'll need to keep a food and exercise diary. You will also have to gather other types of data about yourself and your family. You may have to contact your doctor to answer some of the questions I ask about your health.

Specifically, you will need to know:

- Your most recent blood pressure

- Your cholesterol panel (that includes total cholesterol, LDL cholesterol, HDL cholesterol, and triglycerides)

- Your fasting blood sugar
- What medicines you take and what they are for

You also need to know about the medical problems of your immediate family. Does your mother, father, sister, or brother have high blood pressure, diabetes, or high cholesterol? These chronic diseases tend to run in families, and if your parents or siblings have them, then you are at a higher risk of getting them, too. Does anyone in your immediate family have heart disease such as angina or coronary artery disease, or have any of them had a heart attack? Heart disease runs in families as well, and children of a parent who had a heart attack at a young age (under 45 for a man and under 55 for a woman) are at increased risk themselves of heart disease.

One last piece of information you will need to know about yourself is your waist size. Women who have a waist measuring 35 inches or more and men who have a waist size of 40 inches or more are at increased risk of heart disease and diabetes. They may also have a condition known as metabolic syndrome. The underlying problem of metabolic syndrome is insulin resistance. Essentially this means that the way they digest carbohydrates is abnormal, and this abnormality has a definite impact on the type of diet that would be best for them. When you have all this information available, you will be ready to fill in the questionnaire.

One last word: When you fill out this questionnaire, try to be as honest as possible. The temptation is to lie to yourself—but don't. This is where it matters. Only by knowing yourself can you know the diet that is perfect for you.

## YOUR EATING AND EXERCISE DIARY

So far, I've just been talking about the theories behind this book— what I have learned from my research about diets and appetites and dieters like you. A quick summary:

1. Diets do work—when there is a good match between the diet and the dieter.

2. An individual's optimal diet, your perfect diet, will be determined by many factors: genetic, environmental, personal.

3. The science of satiety—what satisfies you—is still a young field, but it's beginning to reveal that much of what we need to satisfy us is hardwired.

4. Managing your weight can only be successful if you make it easy to do the right thing.

5. Getting out of shape did not happen overnight. Getting back into shape won't either.

6. The best diet for you will be the one that comes closest to fitting you as you are.

That's the theory. Let's get on to the reality. Your first step is to keep a diet diary. Why? Because the perfect diet for you has to be tailored to fit you exactly. And knowing what you eat, when you eat, why you eat is essential in getting that fit. It's like buying a piece of clothing—you can get it off the rack and we often do, but when it's important that the dress or jacket fit perfectly, we usually have to tailor it to make it fit just right. The most important tool a tailor has is his tape measure. That tells him what he needs to know about your body and how to make the garment fit. Your eating and exercise diary will be your tape measure in tailoring your diet.

Look, you know what your body looks like, in general. Maybe you know that you have broad shoulders or long legs, but do you know exactly how broad, how long? Probably not. Same with your diet. You have an idea about what you eat and why you eat it. You have a feeling about how active you are, but you can't really quantify it. Your eating and exercise diary will let you measure what you think you know, but don't know well enough to help you find the diet that is perfect for you.

Of course, you probably think you know what you eat. Be prepared to surprise yourself. There have been lots of studies that show that food recall—that is, just asking people what they eat—is a very poor way to discover the truth about diet. It's not just that people lie, although that may be part of it. It's that most people just don't remember everything they put in their mouths.

Let's look at what the research shows. In a study done a few years ago, researchers had nine women and one man eat a single meal made up of a wide variety of foods. What they chose and how much was eaten was carefully documented by the researchers. The next day the researchers called each of the ten subjects and asked them to remember what they ate in that meal.

They couldn't do it.

They thought they could do it, but when their lists were compared with what they actually ate, it was clear that the subjects weren't nearly as accurate as they thought they were. They could remember some of what they ate, but not everything, and they were just terrible at remembering how much they ate. They couldn't remember even though they had been told before the meal that they would be asked about it the next day. This is only one tiny study, but there have been many that show the same thing—people don't remember what they put into their mouths.

Other researchers have looked for a pattern of what is remembered and what is forgotten about what we eat. They found one. While most of us do a pretty good job of remembering what we eat at mealtimes, snacks were frequently forgotten. It was as if they were never eaten. And when you compare what people ate with what they remember eating, fatty foods and so-called junk foods were most likely to be left off the list.

That's why you need a diary.

When my sister Shelley decided to start this diet, I gave her the whole rap about how she needed to write down everything she ate in order for us to figure out how she should eat to lose weight. She was totally on board, ready to do it, even excited.

When she brought back her diary and her questionnaire, she had a confession to make: She had originally filled out the questionnaire without keeping the diary. She considered herself a reasonable person, someone capable of honestly remembering and reporting what she ate. And she thought that keeping the diary was just too tough and too time consuming. Plus, she was anxious to start the diet.

So she filled out the questionnaire as honestly as she could. And she is a reasonable person. When she looked the questionnaire over, she realized that what she'd written down couldn't possibly represent everything she'd eaten within the past few days because if it did, she'd have just about starved. There simply weren't enough foods on her list.

"I knew I'd left things off my list," she confessed, "but I couldn't remember or even imagine what they were." So she started to keep the diary. It was tough, especially when she had to write down things she felt she "shouldn't have eaten." But she did it.

When she sat down to fill out the questionnaire again, she got an education. She saw what she had left out when she had tried to fill it out without an eating diary. She was surprised, but also interested. "It wasn't just the bad stuff I left off the list, although that was a lot of it." She noticed two types of foods she omitted. The first were foods she didn't think she ate—her example: baked goods. "When I got to that part of the questionnaire the first time, it was a no-brainer. I never eat baked goods—cakes, cookies. Not what I like. But when I kept my diary, I saw that I did eat quite a few baked goods—muffins and biscuits—I even ate a couple of cookies. I couldn't believe it, but there it was in black and white."

Another error she noticed when she compared her first questionnaire with her second was that she was pretty good at remembering what she ate at meals, but snacks just fell off her radar. "If you had asked me if I ate snacks, I would have said that I didn't normally. Actually, keeping this diary made me realize that on one day I ate as much in snacks as I did meals. It blew my mind."

"When I looked at the second questionnaire, it was a little embarrassing, but I knew it was a better picture of my diet than the first one. The first one was what I thought I ate—what I wished I ate. The second one was what I *really* ate."

Keeping a diary isn't just the best reality check for people like Shelley. Scientific research confirms that it's the most reliable method of tracking what we eat. In a British study, 172 men and women were asked to write down everything they ate for a week. Actually, they were asked to do it twice—the second time a year after the first time—in part because the researchers wanted to see how much their diets changed.

Since the participants weren't living in a hospital for all this time, the researchers needed some other way of checking out the accuracy of their eating diaries. So, using the principle that what goes in must come out, they asked the participants to keep all of their urine for one entire day—they did this several times over the course of a year—and the scientists analyzed it for some of the essential components of the diet that would be excreted in the urine. They then compared the foods listed in the diaries with those that showed up in the urine. They found that diaries were pretty good at recording what was eaten. Not 100 percent, but not bad. And much better than asking people what they ate and relying on their memory.

*The Perfect Fit for Peter (lost 90 pounds)*
*I am a victim of the F's: I'm over 40, a father, fit (sort of), failing to make my diet and lifestyle work together and therefore FAT. I got here the easy way. I like to eat, I like to cook, and when I don't think about it I eat too much of what I like.*

*Now I'm not one of those people who get their weight down, only to balloon back up. I'm one of those people who go from overweight to FAT. But now* that I'm on the back side of my forties, my doctor reminded me that at nearly 300 pounds I had the same health risks as people who smoke. Fat people (like me) have heart and lung problems; we're at greater risk for cancer, then there are diabetes, bad knees, bad back, and just plain old bad Karma. I quit smoking over 20 years ago, so why can't I deal with this fat problem?

Well you can't just quit eating, and going hungry doesn't work very well either. That's when I turned to The Perfect Fit Diet. Lisa Sanders has written a book that isn't really a diet and it isn't really one of those lifestyle books either. What this book does is give you a way to look at what you like to eat, when and where you eat it, factor your real life into the equation, and come away with a plan that fits you, lets you eat food you like, and creates an infrastucture for thinking about food in a different, positive way.

The whole diet diary thing was hard. I'm busy, it wasn't easy to make room for just one more thing in an already hectic schedule. But it was more than that. There was a part of me that just didn't want to know. But I've done the diet deal before and I still ended up kissing the 300 mark on the scale so I pulled a Nike—I just did it. And it paid off. I ended up keeping the food diary for close to a month. Writing all that down let me see the stupid stuff I did. I would go down to the Starbucks and get black coffee, but instead of eating the banana in my desk I'd buy a muffin to go with the coffee. I saw that when I was plopped down in front of the TV and watching the game, I'd be getting a beer. Then I'd be getting out the chips and salsa. So just writing stuff down was an important lesson in Peter's Diet 101.

Filling out the questionnaire was a second process. That was a real education on how to think about food. It was really one of the most self-informative and ultimately self-motivating things that I have ever done, and implementing Dr. Sanders's suggestions have allowed me to make some real progress on my long-term goals. I knew I wanted to lose 90 pounds, get my running back up to 30 miles a week, and recapture the energy and focus that I have lost.

That was almost a year ago. Now I'm 90 pounds lighter. I'm running 15 miles a week. Now that my weight is down, I'm sleeping better, and my kids say that I am nicer.

Oh yes, and I'm not hungry. I didn't quit eating the things that I like.

*And I don't have to eat steak or cheeseburgers all the time, or pasta all the time. What is really different is the way I think about my food and what I do with my time. I feel better and I know that I can reach my goals and maintain them because I've found the diet that is the right fit.*

*The book allowed me to put a scientific framework around my eating. The whole science of weight loss—how you lose weight, how the diets work, how your lifestyle can make it hard to lose weight and easy to gain it—made a lot of sense to me. And if you can understand it, you can make changes that work. And that knowledge gives you some wiggle room. Mostly I think I used the book to isolate food that I didn't need—and didn't really want and wouldn't miss. And I figured out what I can do instead of eat. These days when my stress sends me to the refrigerator I know I can take a walk and that'll hold me for a couple of hours.*

*So now I'm down to 188. I started out over 277. I want to get down to 170–175. That's about right for me. The nice thing is that as I sit here today I know I can keep doing it. In fact, it gets easier every week. The longer I do this, the clearer it is to me that this is the right way for me.*

## HOW TO KEEP AN EATING AND EXERCISE DIARY

Enough theory. On to practice.

First, I want you to keep your diary for 4 days. Two days should be weekdays and then a weekend. (There is good evidence that how we eat on the weekends is quite different from how we eat during the week.) And why 4 days? Because that's probably how long it takes to get a flavor for the variation in your diet.

Even careful and honest documentation of everything you put in your mouth won't give you a perfect picture of your diet. Just the act of watching ourselves often changes how we eat. Not really a surprise for many of us. So much of what we eat is done mindlessly—really without our even noticing. Keeping a food diary makes us take notice of exactly what we put in our mouths. And some of those things, now that we're paying attention, we don't really want to eat. So we don't—and that means the food diary isn't completely accurate. It's why we can lose weight just by keeping a diary for a few days.

On the other hand, there's still a lot to be learned from what we do write down. It's really our only tool for understanding the real components of our diet. So flaws and all, keeping a diary is still one of the most useful tools we have in understanding and changing the way we eat.

A few fundamental guidelines about keeping a food diary. First, write down what you eat *at the time you are eating it.* Don't wait until the end of the day to summarize what you ate, because then you are trusting your memory, and as you know, your memory can't be trusted for information like this. Second, keep your diary with you during these 4 days; you never know when you are going to eat or drink something, and you need to write it down as soon as you consume it. Third, if you eat something you can't bring yourself to write down, don't torture yourself—make a mark on the page to indicate missing data and just move on. In this, as in so much of life, the perfect is the enemy of the good.

I have included a 4-day diet diary to help get you started. You can Xerox it or just take the book with you. When you look at the diary you'll see that writing down the food and drink is only one part of the job. You need to keep track of a few other things, too. I call these the Four W's and they are based on the five questions a journalist is supposed to answer in any news story he or she writes. The journalist's questions are Who? What? When? Where? How? Mine are a little different.

When? You will need to write down what time you eat. If you aren't a watch-wearing person, estimate the time. Just the hour is fine. This way you will see when you get hungry, or at least when you eat.

Then, of course, is what? Write down everything you eat and drink.

Then where? Were you at home sitting at the kitchen table? Were you at work? Were you eating out at a restaurant? Were you eating on the run? Did you grab a slice of pizza as you headed to a meeting? Were you in the car, on the way to pick up your child from soccer practice?

Finally, Why? This is the toughest question to answer, but also very important. Sure, sometimes we eat because we are hungry. Often, however, there is a different reason. Many of us eat because of non-hunger cues. Find out what those cues are for you. You might be surprised. Worry or anger are triggers for some. Happiness does it for others. Boredom, stress, nervousness are common triggers. Some of us eat for comfort, some in celebration or as a reward. There are probably as many reasons as there are people, so find out what makes you eat. It will help you lose the weight you want to lose and, just as important, it will help you keep it off.

You will also need to write down your exercise and activity level. Exercise, you know what that is. Just write down what you do, how long you did it, and whether or not you became out of breath while doing it. The activity part isn't so intuitive. Activity is really anything you do that requires you to move in a sustained manner. Watching television or answering e-mail wouldn't count as an activity. A daily activity would be walking up the stairs or taking out the trash. They are things you do at home that require you to move. Housework, gardening, walking to the subway or across a parking lot—those would all count as activities. Write them down as often as you can so that you can see how active you are on a daily basis. I also want you to rate your exertion. If you walked across a parking lot and didn't get out of breath, that's a 1. If you walked up a flight or two of steps and you didn't break a sweat, but you were breathing a little hard, that's a 2. And if you ran to catch your bus, but the driver didn't see you right away so you actually broke out in a sweat, give yourself a 3.

Just a couple of words before I send you off on this task. Keeping a diary is hard work. I can't tell you exactly why, but it is. Part of it, sure, is just doing something you don't normally do in the midst of your very busy day. It's not easy to integrate new practices into your routine. But I suspect it's more than that.

There is something about eating, especially if you weigh more than you want to weigh, something very emotional. And this emotional component makes us reluctant to even *know* about what we eat, much less write it down. I know that even though I don't have a problem with my weight, I have difficulty writing down what I eat. My patients—the ones who are honest, in any case—also acknowledge that it can be tough.

But—and this is important, too—keeping a diary will give you information you didn't have before, information that you can use to change your diet and lifestyle in a way that will fit you perfectly.

Losing weight is not just a matter of eating less, though that is part of it. But you also have to know what to keep. Too often we think of diets only in terms of what we don't eat: I can't eat this and I can't eat that. No wonder they feel like deprivation—the whole thing is about not eating.

A perfect diet is built on foods you do eat—foods you love, foods you need, foods you are going to eat whether they are on your diet or not. A diet diary allows you to see what those foods are. Look, one of the reasons that we keep a diet diary is to find out what we really like. We're afraid of what we really like. We don't want to know. But if you level with yourself and keep track of what you really eat, you will have a much better chance of creating a way to eat that is fun to follow, good to eat, and that will fit you for life.

Making the transformation from periodic dieter to someone who has a diet that works and lasts requires a diet that fits, and the only way to come up with that diet is to understand your body, and your feelings about what you eat and why you eat it.

This diary is the key to all that. Change without direction or understanding—which is all that any off-the-shelf diet has to offer—is change that's going to be hard to maintain. That's why this job of keeping a diary will be the hardest job you'll ever come to love.

## DIET DIARY

# DAY

Workday ☐                              Weekend ☐

This will be the easiest day of the entire diary. You are ready, you have your pen, your diary, your good intentions. I always find that breakfast on day 1 is the easiest meal to document.

### Breakfast:
When (did I eat it)?
What (did I have)?
Where (was I when I ate it)?
Why (did I eat it)?

### A.M. Snacks:
When?
What?
Where?
Why?

### Lunch:
When?
What?
Where?
Why?

### P.M. Snacks:
When?
What?
Where?
Why?

### Dinner:
When?
What?
Where?
Why?

**Bedtime Snacks:**
When?
What?
Where?
Why?

**Beverages:**

| | | | | | | | | |
|---|---|---|---|---|---|---|---|---|
| Water | □ | □ | □ | □ | □ | □ | □ | □ |
| Coffee | □ | □ | □ | □ | □ | □ | □ | □ |
| Tea | □ | □ | □ | □ | □ | □ | □ | □ |
| Milk product | □ | □ | □ | □ | □ | □ | □ | □ |
| Juice | □ | □ | □ | □ | □ | □ | □ | □ |
| Soda | □ | □ | □ | □ | □ | □ | □ | □ |
| Diet soda | □ | □ | □ | □ | □ | □ | □ | □ |
| Other no-cal beverages | □ | □ | □ | □ | □ | □ | □ | □ |
| Alcoholic beverage | □ | □ | □ | □ | □ | □ | □ | □ |

## ACTIVITY DIARY

| Time | Activity or exercise | Duration and level of exertion |
|---|---|---|
| | | Rate exertion on scale of 1–3 |
| | | 1 = no sweat, breathing easily |
| | | 2 = no sweat, breathing hard |
| | | 3 = break a sweat, out of breath |

**Morning**

**Afternoon**

**Evening**

# DAY

Workday ☐                    Weekend ☐

The first day wasn't so bad. You remembered to write just about everything down. Today should also be pretty easy and you will feel good about what you are eating and why. Are you surprised at how often you eat when you are not hungry? Or are you surprised at how often you eat because you are starving? Both of these are common patterns and there are ways of dealing with both.

## Breakfast:
When?
What?
Where?
Why?

## A.M. Snacks:
When?
What?
Where?
Why?

## Lunch:
When?
What?
Where?
Why?

## P.M. Snacks:
When?
What?
Where?
Why?

## Dinner:
When?
What?
Where?
Why?

**Bedtime Snacks:**
When?
What?
Where?
Why?

**Beverages:**

| | | | | | | | | |
|---|---|---|---|---|---|---|---|---|
| Water | □ | □ | □ | □ | □ | □ | □ | □ |
| Coffee | □ | □ | □ | □ | □ | □ | □ | □ |
| Tea | □ | □ | □ | □ | □ | □ | □ | □ |
| Milk product | □ | □ | □ | □ | □ | □ | □ | □ |
| Juice | □ | □ | □ | □ | □ | □ | □ | □ |
| Soda | □ | □ | □ | □ | □ | □ | □ | □ |
| Diet soda | □ | □ | □ | □ | □ | □ | □ | □ |
| Other no-cal beverages | □ | □ | □ | □ | □ | □ | □ | □ |
| Alcoholic beverage | □ | □ | □ | □ | □ | □ | □ | □ |

## ACTIVITY DIARY

| Time | Activity or exercise | Duration and level of exertion |
|---|---|---|
| | | Rate exertion on scale of 1–3 |
| | | 1 = no sweat, breathing easily |
| | | 2 = no sweat, breathing hard |
| | | 3 = break a sweat, out of breath |

**Morning**

**Afternoon**

**Evening**

# DAY

Workday ☐                                    Weekend ☐

My patients tell me this is when it starts feeling hard. They have the challenge of writing down something they don't want to admit—even to themselves. It's okay. You are the only one who will see this. If you don't write it down, then you won't be able to learn from it. Unless you write it down, those foods will just be calories that you are sorry you ate and they won't help you learn about yourself. So yes, it's sometimes hard, but there's a payoff.

**Breakfast:**
When?
What?
Where?
Why?

**A.M. Snacks:**
When?
What?
Where?
Why?

**Lunch:**
When?
What?
Where?
Why?

**P.M. Snacks:**
When?
What?
Where?
Why?

**Dinner:**
When?
What?
Where?
Why?

**Bedtime Snacks:**
When?
What?
Where?
Why?

**Beverages:**

| | | | | | | | | |
|---|---|---|---|---|---|---|---|---|
| Water | ☐ | ☐ | ☐ | ☐ | ☐ | ☐ | ☐ | ☐ |
| Coffee | ☐ | ☐ | ☐ | ☐ | ☐ | ☐ | ☐ | ☐ |
| Tea | ☐ | ☐ | ☐ | ☐ | ☐ | ☐ | ☐ | ☐ |
| Milk product | ☐ | ☐ | ☐ | ☐ | ☐ | ☐ | ☐ | ☐ |
| Juice | ☐ | ☐ | ☐ | ☐ | ☐ | ☐ | ☐ | ☐ |
| Soda | ☐ | ☐ | ☐ | ☐ | ☐ | ☐ | ☐ | ☐ |
| Diet soda | ☐ | ☐ | ☐ | ☐ | ☐ | ☐ | ☐ | ☐ |
| Other no-cal beverages | ☐ | ☐ | ☐ | ☐ | ☐ | ☐ | ☐ | ☐ |
| Alcoholic beverage | ☐ | ☐ | ☐ | ☐ | ☐ | ☐ | ☐ | ☐ |

## ACTIVITY DIARY

| Time | Activity or exercise | Duration and level of exertion |
|---|---|---|
| | | Rate exertion on scale of 1–3 |
| | | 1 = no sweat, breathing easily |
| | | 2 = no sweat, breathing hard |
| | | 3 = break a sweat, out of breath |

**Morning**

**Afternoon**

**Evening**

# DAY

Workday □                    Weekend □

As you write down each of the foods you eat today, try to quantify how much you enjoyed it. The automatic answer is "I love them all," and maybe like a mother with her children you did love each and every bite in its own way. Most people however eat on autopilot. How much of what you ate did you really enjoy and how much did you eat because it was there? Which of the foods that you ate could you live without and which were essential?

**Breakfast:**
When?
What?
Where?
Why?

**A.M. Snacks:**
When?
What?
Where?
Why?

**Lunch:**
When?
What?
Where?
Why?

**P.M. Snacks:**
When?
What?
Where?
Why?

**Dinner:**
When?
What?
Where?
Why?

**Bedtime Snacks:**
When?
What?
Where?
Why?

**Beverages:**

| | | | | | | | | |
|---|---|---|---|---|---|---|---|---|
| Water | □ | □ | □ | □ | □ | □ | □ | □ |
| Coffee | □ | □ | □ | □ | □ | □ | □ | □ |
| Tea | □ | □ | □ | □ | □ | □ | □ | □ |
| Milk product | □ | □ | □ | □ | □ | □ | □ | □ |
| Juice | □ | □ | □ | □ | □ | □ | □ | □ |
| Soda | □ | □ | □ | □ | □ | □ | □ | □ |
| Diet soda | □ | □ | □ | □ | □ | □ | □ | □ |
| Other no-cal beverages | □ | □ | □ | □ | □ | □ | □ | □ |
| Alcoholic beverage | □ | □ | □ | □ | □ | □ | □ | □ |

## ACTIVITY DIARY

| Time | Activity or exercise | Duration and level of exertion |
|---|---|---|
| | | Rate exertion on scale of 1–3 |
| | | 1 = no sweat, breathing easily |
| | | 2 = no sweat, breathing hard |
| | | 3 = break a sweat, out of breath |

**Morning**

**Afternoon**

**Evening**

# 5 CHAPTER
## YOUR PERFECT FIT QUESTIONNAIRE

THIS QUESTIONNAIRE IS THE map to your perfect fit diet. I'm going to ask you questions about what you eat, how you eat it, and how you feel about it. I'm going to ask you about how you have dieted in the past: what worked, what didn't, what you craved, why you stopped. I'm going to ask you about your parents' health and yours, too. And I'm going to ask you about the activity in your life.

There are a lot of questions simply because how we eat, how we exercise, and how our bodies react are complicated and shaped by many forces. This test will help you figure out your Perfect Fit Diet by trying to take as many of those complex factors into consideration as possible.

Let's do a quick inventory of what you will need to complete this questionnaire. Check these off as you collect the information.

___ You have your food diary that reports everything you have eaten or drunk for a total of 4 days and your 4-day activity diary.*

___ You've called your doctor and gotten your blood pressure, fasting glucose, and cholesterol profile.

___ You've called your parents or siblings to find out what types of chronic illness they've had.

___ You have a tape measure to determine your waist size.

As you fill out the questionnaire, you will notice that it's broken up into sections. Each set of questions has been developed to evaluate a specific aspect of your diet and your preferences. You're going to have to keep track of your answers, so I have left spaces for you to fill in with your answer. You will need to total your score at the end of each section. If you can't bring yourself to write in a book, get a piece of lined paper and number it from 1 to 83 and record your answers there. Or better yet, photocopy the model answer sheet I have included just after the questionnaire.

At the end of each section, there is a little grading system for it. Most sections will give you two types of answers: One will be part of a cumulative score that directs you to one of the three main diet plans. At the very end of each section you will see a line where you can mark which diet that part of the questionnaire recommends for you. You will give yourself a point in either the Counting Carbohydrates category, the Counting Calories category, or the Counting Fats category. When you finish, you will tally up your points for each diet, and the one that gets the most will be the one most likely to suit you perfectly.

*If you haven't been able to keep a diary, do not despair—there is a way to complete the questionnaire without it. Simply follow the directions for the Jump-Start version, and we can go from there.

The other type of answer will be a score that will help you customize your diet based on specific aspects of your food preferences, family and medical history, and dieting history. You can do the sections one at a time and score yourself at the end of each, or you can plow through to the end and then calculate your two scores.

## HOW TO CHEAT

Some of you (and you know who you are) will not be able to make yourself fill out the food diary. Maybe you're too impatient to wait the 4 days. Maybe you tried but found that writing all this down was simply too hard or too loaded with emotional baggage. For whatever reason, there is a population of readers who choose to fill out the questionnaire without the food diary. What has happened in the past is that these folks answer the questions that were supposed to be from the food diary based on their best guess about what they ate and drank. And you know that just doesn't work.

This questionnaire is designed to pick up small differences in the way people eat, drink, and snack. A food diary gives you the best chance to pick up on those differences. Relying on memory doesn't do it—and at this point I hope it's clear why.

I wasn't sure what to do about the folks who don't want to keep a food diary—I wished there was some way to change their minds. And then, I had dinner with a friend, Cam. She confessed that she couldn't keep the diary, either. I laughed and told her that she's not alone, explaining that several readers had told me the same thing. "What should I do?" I asked her.

"Find room for me and readers like me in your book," she challenged. "You're the one who says you have to make it easy to do the right thing. Physician, heal your book!"

Okay, Cam, I have.

For all of you who, like Cam, simply cannot fill out the food diary, you can now Jump-Start your diet. The first seven questions of the questionnaire are based on the food diary—simply skip that section. For you, the questionnaire will start at question 8. This means that the most you will have is 10 points divided among the three diet categories.

## THE QUESTIONNAIRE

Please answer the following questions. Some will ask you to look at your food diary; others will be based on what you know about yourself. Keep in mind that there are no right or wrong answers; only *your* answers. This isn't about whether the way you eat is healthy; this questionnaire is about how you eat, period.

> *"From principles is derived probability, but truth or certainty is obtained only from facts."* —Nathaniel Hawthorne

> *"Just the facts, ma'am."* —Joe Friday, *Dragnet*

# THE PERFECT FIT QUESTIONNAIRE

## PART 1: FOOD PREFERENCES

1.  Are you a Carnimore? Over the course of your 4-day diary, how many servings of these foods did you eat?

    | | |
    |---|---|
    | Chicken or other poultry | _____ |
    | Beef or veal | _____ |
    | Pork | _____ |
    | Lamb or other meat | _____ |
    | Fish or other seafood | _____ |
    | Eggs | _____ |

If you ate more than 5 servings of these foods, chances are you are a Carnimore. For details on how to work with your carnivorous self, see page 231. In the meantime, give yourself 1 point in the carb-counting row and one in the calorie-counting row. If you ate more than 8 servings of these foods, give yourself 2 points in the carb-counting plan and one in the calorie-counting plan.

Diet plan:

Count carbs _____

Count cals _____

Count fat _____

2.  Are you a Milk Mavin? Over the course of your 4-day food diary, how many servings of these foods did you eat?

    | | |
    |---|---|
    | Milk (½ cup is 1 serving; milk in your coffee is ½ serving) | _____ |
    | Half-and-half or cream (½ cup is 1 serving; the cream in your coffee is ½ serving) | _____ |
    | Butter | _____ |

Cheese          _____

Yogurt          _____

Ice cream        _____

If you ate more than 6 servings of these foods, then you fit my criteria for a Milk Mavin. For details on how to work with this aspect of your diet, see page 242. In the meantime, give yourself 1 point for the carb-counting plan and 1 point for the calorie-counting plan.

Diet plan:                              Count carbs _____

                                         Count cals _____

                                         Count fat _____

3. Are you a VegeCarian? Over the course of your 4-day food diary, how many servings of these foods did you have?

Green salad          _____

Green veggies (not salad)        _____

Red, yellow, purple, white, or orange veggies
(don't count potatoes here, I ask about them later)    _____

Fruit of any type        _____

Fruit or vegetable juice
(each small glass equals ½ serving)    _____

Frozen fruit bars (each bar equals ½ serving)    _____

If you ate 8 or more servings, you're a VegeCarian. For details on how to work with this in your diet, see page 245. In the meantime, give yourself 1 point in the fat-counting row and 1 point in the calorie-counting row. If you ate more than 10 servings, give yourself 2 points for the fat-counting plan, and 1 point for the calorie-counting plan. If you ate fewer than 8 servings, give yourself 1 point for the carbohydrate-counting plan.

Diet plan:                              Count carbs _____

                                        Count cals _____

                                        Count fat _____

4.  Are you a Starch Stealer? Over the course of your 4-day food diary,
    how many servings of these foods did you have?

    Potatoes                                                _____

    Rice                                                    _____

    Pasta                                                   _____

    Bread (count a sandwich as 2 servings)                  _____

    Baked goods (crackers, cookies, muffins,
        bagels, cakes, donuts)                              _____

    Cereal (hot or cold)                                    _____

    Pizza                                                   _____

    Chips                                                   _____

If you had 8 or more servings, you are a Starch Stealer. For more
about this, see page 252. Then give yourself 1 point for the fat-
counting plan and 1 for the calorie-counting plan. If you had 12 or
more servings, then give yourself 2 points for the fat-counting
plan and 1 for the calorie-counting plan. If you had fewer than 8
servings in your diary, give yourself 1 point for the carb-counting
plan.

            Diet plan:                  Count carbs _____

                                        Count cals _____

                                        Count fat _____

5. Are you a Sweets Eater? How many servings of these foods have you
   had over the past 4 days?

   Sweet baked goods (cookies, cakes, muffins, pies)        _____

   Chocolate (candy, ice cream, or drinks)                  _____

Candy (not including the chocolate
   you just told me about) _____

Soda (including diet soda) _____

Juice or other sweet drinks _____

Fruit (leave out the pastries and other fruit-based
   sweets you've already counted in this section) _____

If you had 6 or more servings of these foods during the period covered by your food diary, then there's a good chance you are a Sweets Eater. You can work with this; see page 257 for details on how. But for now, give yourself 1 point for the fat-counting plan and 1 for the calorie-counting plan. If you had 10 servings or more, give yourself 2 points for the fat-counting plan. If you had fewer than 6, give yourself 1 point for the carb-counting plan.

Diet plan:                          Count carbs _____

                                    Count cals _____

                                    Count fat _____

6. Are you a Junk-Food Junkie? How many servings of these foods did you have over the past 4 days?

Fast-food burgers _____

Fast-food French fries _____

Fast-food chicken (any type) _____

Fast-food tacos, burritos _____

Fast-food milkshake _____

Fast-food donut or muffin _____

Pizza _____

Chips (any type) _____

Candy (any type) _____

Cookies (any type) _____

If you had 6 or more servings of these foods in your 4-day diet diary, then there's a good chance you are a Junk-Food Junkie. Although the media may have convinced you that fast foods are the source of all evil—or at least the cause of our national expanding waistline—there are ways of incorporating these foods into a diet that works for you. See page 266 for details on how to do this. But for now, give yourself 1 point for the carb-counting plan and 1 for the calorie-counting plan. If you had 9 servings or more, give yourself 2 points for the carb-counting plan. If you had fewer than 2, give yourself 1 point for the fat-counting plan.

Diet plan:

Count carbs _____

Count cals _____

Count fat _____

7. Do you drink enough liquids in a day or are you a Waterless Wonder? How many servings of these drinks have you recorded in your 4-day food diary?

Water (flavored or not) _____

Soda or pop (diet or regular) _____

Fruit or vegetable juices _____

Tea _____

Milk products _____

Total _____

Not all drinks count toward your total score. Do not count coffee, beer, or other alcoholic drinks. (Don't even count the mixers.)

If you had fewer than 6 servings of these drinks over the course of your 4-day diary, you are parched—a real Waterless Wonder. No matter what diet you are on, you're going to need to drink more than that! See page 275 on how much is enough. And give yourself 1 point for the fat-counting plan.

If you had more than 6 but fewer than 16 drinks over the course of your 4-day diary, give yourself 1 point for the fat-counting plan, and 1 for the calories-counting plan. You too should turn to p. 275 to find out more about what water can do for you.

If you had more than 16 drinks over the course of your 4 days, congratulations. You are doing a pretty good job keeping your body well watered and your kidneys well lubricated. Give yourself 1 point in each of the three diet categories.

Diet plan:

Count carbs _____

Count cals _____

Count fat _____

## Simple PROP Test

(Answer these questions based on what you know about yourself and your preferences.)

8.  I find brussels sprouts:                    _____

    a. Very tasty

    b. Moderately tasty

    c. Moderately distasteful

    d. Very distasteful

9.  I find broccoli:                    _____

    a. Very tasty

    b. Moderately tasty

    c. Moderately distasteful

    d. Very distasteful

10. I find saccharine:                    _____

    a. Very sweet

    b. Moderately sweet

    c. Sweet but moderately bitter

d. Sweet but very bitter

e. I don't like saccharine, but I don't know why

11. I find grapefruit (without sugar): _____

a. Very tasty

b. Moderately tasty

c. Moderately distasteful

d. Very distasteful

12. I do not like foods that taste even a little bit bitter. _____

a. True

b. False

13. I often find desserts too sweet to enjoy. _____

a. True

b. False

14. I do not like foods that are very rich. _____

a. True

b. False

15. Fried foods often seem too oily for me to enjoy. _____

a. True

b. False

Scoring 8–11: Give yourself 1 point for every *a*, 5 points for every *b*, 10 points for every *c*, 20 points for every *d* or *e*.

Scoring 12–15: Give yourself 0 points for every *false*; give yourself 10 points for every *true*.

If you have a score of 40 or greater, you may be a PROP taster. If your score is greater than 70, you may even be a Supertaster. For details on this aspect of your preferences, see page 284.

If your score is 40 or greater, give yourself 1 point for the calorie-counting plan and 1 for the carb-counting plan.

If your score is less than 40, give yourself 1 point for the fat-counting plan.

Diet plan:

Count carbs _____

Count cals _____

Count fat _____

# PART 2: DIETING HISTORY

## What Makes You Feel Full?

16. The most successful diet I have tried was:          _____
    (Pick as many as apply.)

    a. Low fat

    b. Low calorie

    c. Low carb

    d. None of the above

17. The most common reason for quitting a diet was:          _____
    (Pick as many as apply.)

    a. Not enough food—a feeling that I hadn't had enough to eat at the meal

    b. Boredom with the foods I was "allowed" to eat

    c. Hunger between meals

    d. None of the above

18. When dieting, what I crave most is:          _____
    (Pick as many as apply.)

    a. Bread, pasta, or sweets

    b. Whatever I'm not allowed to eat

c. Meat, cheese, butter

d. None of the above

19. Select any of the following statements
about how you eat:                                    _____
(Pick as many as apply.)

a. I need to eat a lot of food to really feel full.

b. I sometimes find myself standing in front of the refrigerator trying to figure out what I am hungry for. If I find it and eat it, I will be satisfied.

c. When I snack, I would rather have a piece of cheese than a piece of fruit.

d. None of these statements are true about me.

20. Select any of the statements about how you eat:      _____
(Pick as many as apply.)

a. A really good meal is one in which I can pile my plate high with food.

b. I prefer a meal composed of several foods to one consisting of any single food.

c. A meal of fresh fruits and vegetables doesn't fill me up.

d. None of these statements are true about me.

21. Select any of the statements about how you eat:      _____
(Pick as many as apply.)

a. I could cut back on eating meat, cheese, and butter, as long as I could eat a large quantity of other foods.

b. Although neither is easy, I would rather restrict my portion size than limit the types of foods I can eat.

c. I don't mind eating a limited variety of foods so long as I don't have to limit my portion size.

d. None of these statements is true about me.

22. I can't imagine life without: _____
    (Choose only one food group containing the food you love.)

    a. Carbs: bread and baked goods, sweets, pasta

    b. Combos: chips, ice cream, French fries, donuts

    c. Fats: butter, cheese, bacon, fried chicken

    Scoring 16–22: To score this section, please tally up:
    How often did you choose the answer marked *a*? _____
    How often did you choose the answer marked *b*? _____
    How often did you choose the answer marked *c*? _____
    How often did you choose the answer marked *d*? _____

If you chose more than 4 *a*'s, give yourself 2 points for the fat-counting plan. Chances are that you take your satiety cues from the volume of food you eat. You can read more about that on page 182.

If you chose more than 4 *b*'s, give yourself 2 points for the calorie-counting plan. You take your cues to stop eating from the variety in your diet. You can read more about this on page 149.

If you chose more than 4 *c*'s, give yourself 2 points for the carb-counting plan. Your satiety signals are loudest when you eat rich foods containing protein and fat.

If you chose more than 4 *d*'s, then you may have cues to stop eating that I haven't asked about. Your satiety signals may not have been described yet. The science of what makes us stop eating is still very young. You should try to figure out what makes you feel full and well fed. A diet that features these foods will allow you to eat less without feeling hungry or deprived. If nothing ever makes you feel satisfied or full, you should at least consider the possibility that you have an eating disorder.

Finally, if you ended up evenly divided among the three categories, you get your satiety cues from more than one of these aspects. Give yourself 1 point in each of the diet plan categories.

Diet plan:

Count carbs _____

Count cals _____

Count fat _____

## How Dieting Changes the Way You Eat

(If you have never dieted before, you should skip this section.)

23. I have dieted: _____

   a. Occasionally

   b. Frequently

   c. All the time

24. In general, these diets were: _____

   a. Very successful. (I lost weight and kept it all off for greater than 6 months.)

   b. Transiently successful. (I lost weight but gained it back within 6 months.)

   c. Never successful. (I never lost any significant weight.)

25. When I see someone eating something, it often makes me want to eat that, even if I am not hungry. _____

   a. Never

   b. Once or twice a week

   c. Frequently

26. Which sentence describes how you feel while dieting? (Mark as many as apply.) _____

   a. I sometimes eat less at a meal than I would like to eat.

   b. When I have eaten the amount of food I think I should eat, I am pretty good about not eating anymore.

   c. When I eat something that is not on my diet, it's hard to get back on track.

   d. I feel great when dieting.

27. My weight has changed by more than 20 pounds over the past year. (If you were pregnant in the past year, count the previous year's weight.) _____

    T  F

28. I'm a yo-yo dieter. _____

    T  F

29. When I eat something that is not on my diet, I often find it difficult to resume my diet. _____

    T  F

30. When I see someone overeat, I have a tendency to overeat, too.

    _____

    T  F

Scoring 23–30: For the multiple choice questions, give yourself 1 point for every *a*, 5 for every *b*, and 10 for every *c*. Give yourself 0 points for *d*'s. For the true/false questions, give yourself 0 points for every *false* and 10 points for every *true*.

   Total for 23–30: _____

   If you have a score greater than 30, then some of your dieting behaviors may be contributing to your inability to manage your weight. For more information on that, see page 301.

## Binge Eating Disorder

31. Which of the following responses best describes your overall eating patterns? _____

    a. I never have trouble with overeating.

    b. I sometimes feel that I eat too much during particular eating episodes.

    c. I occasionally eat within a 2-hour period what I and most people would consider an unusually large amount of food.

d. I quite often eat within a 2-hour period what I and most people would consider an unusually large amount of food.

If you answered *a* or *b*, then you are unlikely to have a binge eating disorder, and you can skip to the next section.

32. When you eat a large amount of food within a 2-hour period, how often do you feel as if you cannot stop eating or control what or how much you eat? _____

   a. Never

   b. Rarely

   c. Occasionally

   d. Always

33. How do you feel when this type of eating takes place? _____
   (Pick as many as apply.)

   a. My eating is more rapid than usual.

   b. I eat until I feel uncomfortably full.

   c. The eating occurs when I am not feeling physically hungry.

   d. When I experience this eating behavior, I do it alone, because I am embarrassed by the amount of food I eat.

   e. After my eating episode, I feel disgusted with myself, depressed, or guilty for overeating.

34. How often have you engaged in this type of behavior over the past 6 months? _____

   a. Less than once a month

   b. Once a month to a few times a month

   c. A few times a month to two times a week

   d. Two times a week

   e. Daily

35. When you eat large amounts of food at one time and feel as though you cannot stop eating, how certain are you that you can control these episodes of eating? _____

   a. Extremely certain

   b. Quite certain

   c. Somewhat certain

   d. Slightly certain

   e. Not at all certain

36. How upset were you that you were not able to control what or how much you were eating? _____

   a. Not at all upset

   b. Slightly upset

   c. Somewhat upset

   d. Quite upset

Scoring 21–36: Give yourself 1 point for every *a*, 2 for every *b*, 3 for every *c*, 4 for every *d*, and 5 for every *e*.

Total: _____

If your score is less than 11, you don't have an eating disorder. If your score is 11 or higher, you are at risk of having one and should discuss this with your doctor before starting on any diet. (See page 303 for more information.)

# PART 3: MEDICAL HISTORY

## Your Own History

37. Mark each statement about your medical history that is true for you.

   a. I smoke cigarettes. _____

b. I have high total cholesterol (greater than 200 mg/dl). _____

c. I have high LDL cholesterol (greater than 160 mg/dl). _____

d. I have low HDL cholesterol (less than 50 mg/dl). _____

e. I have high triglycerides (greater than 150 mg/dl). _____

f. My doctor has prescribed medicine for my cholesterol. _____

g. *I've never had my cholesterol tested.* _____

h. I have diabetes. _____

i. *I have never been tested for diabetes.* _____

j. I have high blood pressure (greater than 120/80 mm Hg). _____

k. *I have never had my blood pressure taken.* _____

l. I have heart disease (angina, coronary artery disease, history of heart attack). _____

m. I am a man. _____

n. I am older than 54 years old. _____

If you are under the age of 25 and marked any of the statements written in *italics* that say you never had your cholesterol or your blood pressure measured, or have never been tested for diabetes, count those statements as 0 and continue.

If you are 25 or older and marked any of the questions in *italics*, you should contact your doctor for further evaluation of your cardiac risk factors.

Give yourself 1 point for each true statement not in italics in the list above.

Total: _____

If you have a score of 3 or greater, chances are that you are at increased risk of heart disease and should consult your doctor before starting any diet or exercise regimen. For further information on what these cardiac risk factors mean, turn to page 305.

If you have a score of 3 or greater, give yourself 1 point for the fat-counting plan.

If you have a score ranging from 0 to 2, give yourself 1 point for both the carb-counting plan and calorie-counting plan.

Diet plan:                    Count carbs _____

                              Count cals _____

                              Count fat _____

## Your Family History

38. Mark each statement about your medical history that is true for your family. If you don't have information on your parents, you can skip this section.

    a. My father had a heart attack before he was 45.        _____

    b. My mother had a heart attack before she was 55.       _____

    c. My mother or father has had coronary bypass surgery.  _____

    d. My mother or father has diabetes.                     _____

    e. My mother or father has high blood pressure.          _____

    f. My mother or father has high cholesterol.             _____

Give yourself 1 point for every statement you marked.

Total: _____

These are also cardiac risk factors. If you have a score of 3 or greater, give yourself 1 point for the fat-counting plan. If you have a score ranging from 0 to 2, give yourself 1 point for both the carb-counting and calorie-counting plan.

Diet plan:                    Count carbs _____

                              Count cals _____

                              Count fat _____

# Metabolic Syndrome

39. Mark each statement that is true for you.

   a. I have a low HDL cholesterol (less than 40 mg/dl for men, less than 50 mg/dl for women). _____

   b. I have high triglycerides (greater than 150 mg/dl). _____

   c. I carry much of my extra weight around my middle (waist 40 inches or greater for men, 35 inches or greater for women). _____

   d. I have high blood pressure (higher than 120/80mm Hg) or am taking medicine for high blood pressure. _____

   e. I have diabetes or am taking medicine for diabetes. _____

Give yourself 1 point for every statement you marked.

   Total: _____

If you have a score of 3 or more, you have metabolic syndrome, and you can read about what this means in terms of how you should eat on page 317. Also give yourself 2 points for the carb-counting plan and 1 point for the calorie-counting plan.

If you answered true to two questions and don't know your HDL cholesterol or your triglycerides or haven't been tested for diabetes, you should discuss your risk with your doctor and ask him to test you for metabolic syndrome.

If you have a score greater than 0 but less than 3, you do not have metabolic syndrome, but you are at risk for it. You also should read about this condition and the way to eat to lower your risk of developing the condition. Also give yourself 1 point for the calorie-counting plan.

If you have a score of 0, then give yourself 1 point for the fat-counting plan.

   Diet plan:                 Count carbs _____

                              Count cals _____

                              Count fat _____

# PART 4: FAMILY HERITAGE

## How You Are Shaped by Nature

40. In my family:
    (Mark all that apply; if none are true, leave blank.) _____

    a. I am the only one who is overweight.

    b. My mother is overweight.

    c. My father is overweight.

    d. One or more of my siblings are overweight.


41. I am overweight in the same way as my:
    (Mark all that apply.) _____

    a. Mother

    b. Father

    c. Siblings

    d. Grandparents


42. Mark each statement that is true for you or your family: _____

    a. I have a lot of nervous energy and need to move almost all the time.

    b. One or both of my parents have a lot of nervous energy and need to move almost all the time.

    c. No one in my family likes vegetables.

    d. Everyone in my family likes meat.

    e. When I see someone overeating, I am more likely to overeat as well.

    f. I have noticed that others in my family overeat when they are around someone who is overeating.

Scoring 40–42: Give yourself 1 point for every marked answer.
    Total: _____

If you have a score of 5 or more, genetics are probably playing an important role in your weight. For more information on how your genes can affect your weight, see page 00.

## How You Are Shaped by Nurture

43. Mark each statement that is true for you: _____
    (Mark all that apply.)

    a. When I was growing up, food was used as a reward.

    b. When I was growing up, food was used as a form of medicine for physical or emotional injuries.

    c. When I was growing up, the meals I ate with my family were the best part of the day.

    d. When I was growing up, cleaning your plate was a must at the dinner table.

44. When I was growing up, meals were characterized by: _____
    (Mark only one answer.)

    a. Just the right amount of food

    b. Too much food

    c. Too little food

    d. Occasions when members of my family went hungry because there wasn't enough food

45. When I was growing up: _____
    (Mark only one answer.)

    a. My family frequently engaged in sports or other physical activities together (hiking, bicycling, gardening, etc.).

    b. My family occasionally engaged in sports or other physical activities together.

    c. My parents weren't active but encouraged and helped me participate in sports or other physical activities.

    d. My parents discouraged my participation in sports or other physical activities.

46. When I was growing up:  _____
    (Mark only one answer.)

    a. I was involved in sports and other physical activities daily.

    b. I frequently participated in sports or other physical activities.

    c. I occasionally participated in sports or other physical activities.

    d. I rarely participated in sports or other physical activities.

47. When I was growing up:  _____
    (Mark only one answer.)

    a. I watched television less than 4 hours per week.

    b. I watched television between 4 and 8 hours per week.

    c. I watched television between 8 and 12 hours per week.

    d. I watched television more than 12 hours per week.

For question 43, give yourself 1 point for every marked answer. For questions 44–47, give yourself 1 point for every *a*, 5 for every *b*, 10 for every *c*, and 20 for every *d*.

    Total: _____

If you have a score of 25 or more, your experiences growing up may be contributing to your difficulty of managing your weight now. For more information on this, turn to page 327.

# PART 5: HOW YOU EAT

## Eating Habits

48. I skip breakfast:  _____

    a. Never or rarely

    b. Once or twice a week

    c. Several times a week

    d. I always skip breakfast.

49. I skip lunch: _____

   a. Never or rarely

   b. Once or twice a week

   c. Several times a week

   d. I always skip lunch.

50. I skip dinner: _____

   a. Never or rarely

   b. Once or twice a week

   c. Several times a week

   d. I always skip dinner.

51. When I sit down to a meal, I feel like I'm starving: _____

   a. Never or rarely

   b. Once or twice a week

   c. Often

   d. Always

52. I snack before lunch: _____

   a. Never or rarely

   b. Once or twice a week

   c. Several times a week

   d. Most days

53. I snack between lunch and dinner: _____

   a. Never or rarely

   b. Once or twice a week

   c. Several times a week

   d. Most days

54. I snack after dinner:                                    _____

    a. Never or rarely

    b. Once or twice a week

    c. Several times a week

    d. Most days


55. I am so hungry at some point during the day
    that I feel as if I have to eat something right away:     _____

    a. Never or rarely

    b. Once or twice a week

    c. Several times a week

    d. Most days

Scoring 48–55: Give yourself 1 point for every *a*, 5 for every *b*, 10 for every *c*, and 20 for every *d*.

Total: _____

If you have a score of less than 10, then you have pretty good eating habits, and the foods you eat are keeping you full from meal to meal.

If you have a score of 10 to 40, your eating habits may be contributing to your difficulty achieving and maintaining your target weight. For information on what we know about effective eating habits, see page 330.

If you have a score greater than 40, then how you structure your eating is making it difficult to achieve and maintain your target weight. You should check out how this is affecting your weight— turn to page 330.

## Emotional Eating

Answer these questions based on your diet diary as well as what you know about yourself.

56. I eat because of boredom: _____

   a. Never

   b. Occasionally, but rarely more than once a week

   c. Frequently—at least twice a week

   d. Daily

57. I eat because I feel stressed: _____

   a. Never

   b. Occasionally, but rarely more than once a week

   c. Frequently—at least twice a week

   d. Daily

58. I eat because of an unpleasant emotion, such as
    anger or depression: _____

   a. Never

   b. Occasionally, but rarely more than once a week

   c. Frequently—at least twice a week

   d. Daily

59. I eat as a reward: _____

   a. Never

   b. Occasionally, but rarely more than once a week

   c. Frequently—at least twice a week

   d. Daily

60. I eat for comfort: _____

   a. Never

   b. Occasionally, but rarely more than once a week

   c. Frequently—at least twice a week

   d. Daily

61. I eat while watching television: _____

   a. Never

   b. Occasionally, but rarely more than once a week

   c. Frequently—at least twice a week

   d. Daily

62. I eat while engaged in another activity,
    such as reading or driving: _____

   a. Never

   b. Occasionally, but rarely more than once a week

   c. Frequently—at least twice a week

   d. Daily

63. I eat out of habit (popcorn at the movies—whether you
    are hungry or not, candy from the workplace candy bowl,
    whether you are hungry or not): _____

   a. Never

   b. Occasionally, but rarely more than once a week

   c. Frequently—at least twice a week

   d. Daily

Scoring 56–63: Give yourself 1 point for every *a*, 5 for every *b*, 10 for every *c*, and 20 for every *d*.

Total: _____

If your score is less than 15, you have pretty good eating habits and usually do not use food to address a non-hunger need. Good for you.

If you have a score of 15 to 40, then emotional eating or habitual eating may be contributing to your difficulty achieving and maintaining your target weight.

If your score is greater than 40, eating when you are not hungry, is making it difficult for you to achieve and maintain your target weight. To learn about emotional or habitual eating, see page 338.

# PART 6: LIFESTYLE

## Eating Out

(Some of these answers draw on your food diary. If you didn't keep a diary, answer all questions based on your average week.)

64. In my food diary, I ate out at a restaurant:  _____

    a. Never

    b. Once

    c. Twice

    d. More than twice

65. In an average week, I eat out:  _____

    a. Never or rarely

    b. Once

    c. 2 to 4 times

    d. More than 4 times

66. In my food diary, I ate at a fast-food restaurant:  _____

    a. Never

    b. Once

    c. Twice

    d. More than twice

67. In an average week, I am most likely to stop at a fast-food restaurant for a meal or snack:  _____

    a. Never or rarely

    b. Once

    c. 2 to 4 times

    d. More than 4 times

68. In an average week I eat my desk: _____

    a. Never

    b. Once

    c. Twice

    d. More than twice

69. I grab something quick to eat from a vending machine: _____

    a. Frequently (3 to 4 times a week)

    b. Twice a week

    c. Occasionally, but at least once a week

    d. Never

70. In an average week, I bring my lunch to work: _____

    a. Frequently (3 to 4 times a week)

    b. Twice a week

    c. Occasionally, but at least once a week

    d. Never

71. In an average week I eat while driving or in a car: _____

    a. Never

    b. Once

    c. Twice

    d. More than twice

72. Choose the statement that best describes the ways in
which your work and other obligations affect how
you eat: _____

    a. I work at home and so can eat what I like, when I'm hungry.

    b. I work outside the home but I am usually able to stop and eat
lunch or a snack when I get hungry.

c. I work outside the home and my schedule is pretty regular, but I end up going 5–6 hours between meals and I can't snack.

d. My obligations make it impossible for me to eat on regular schedule.

Scoring 64–72: Give yourself 1 point for every *a*, 5 for every *b*, 10 for every *c*, and 20 for every *d*.

Total: _____

If you have a score of 30 or more, where you are eating may be having a big impact on your ability to lose weight or maintain your weight loss. Turn to page 346 for some tips on how to work with these common problems of modern life.

If you have a score of less than 30, then you are able to maintain pretty good control of what you eat, so give yourself 1 point for each of the three diet plans.

If you scored between 30 and 50 points, you eat out of the house often enough so that a diet that requires you to keep track of fat will be hard to follow. Give yourself 1 point for the carb-counting plan and for the calorie-counting plan.

If you have more than 50 points, you eat out a lot, so give yourself 1 point for the carb-counting plan.

Diet plan:

Count carbs _____

Count cals _____

Count fat _____

## Daily Activity

Answer these questions based on your activity diary.

73. Most days, I climbed stairs: _____

a. Never or rarely

b. 1 or 2 flights per day

c. 3 to 5 flights per day

d. More than 5 flights per day

74. Most days I walked: _____

a. Less than 1 block per day

b. 1 to 2 blocks per day

c. More than 2 blocks but less than 10 blocks per day

d. 10 or more blocks per day

75. Which best describes how you got to
your workplace? _____

a. I drove to work and parked nearby.

b. I drove to work, parked, and walked a block or so to work.

c. I took public transportation to work.

d. I walked or bicycled to work.

76. Which best describes how much time you
spent sitting (both at work and at home)? _____

a. I sit more than 12 hours per day.

b. I sit between 8 and 12 hours per day.

c. I sit between 4 and 8 hours per day.

d. I sit less than 4 hours per day.

77. Which best describes how much time per
week you spent doing housework
(cleaning, cooking, laundry, etc.)? _____

a. Less than 1 hour per week

b. Between 1 and 3 hours per week

c. Between 3 and 6 hours per week

d. More than 6 hours per week

78. Which best describes how much time per
    week you spent working in your yard or garden?          _____

    a. Are you kidding? Who has the time or the space
       for a garden?

    b. Less than 2 hours per week

    c. Between 2 and 5 hours per week

    d. More than 5 hours per week

79. Which best describes how much time each day
    you spent watching television?                          _____

    a. More than 5 hours per day

    b. Between 3 and 5 hours per day

    c. Between 1 and 3 hours per day

    d. Less than 1 hour per day

80. Which best describes how much time each day you
    spent in your car?                                      _____

    a. More than 5 hours per day

    b. Between 3 and 5 hours per day

    c. Between 1 and 3 hours per day

    d. Less than 1 hour per day

81. Most weeks I work outside the home                      _____
    (include volunteer work as well as work for which you are paid):

    a. More than 50 hours per week

    b. Between 40 and 50 hours per week

    c. Between 25 and 40 hours per week

    d. Less than 25 hours per week

Scoring 73–81: Give yourself 1 point for every *a*, 5 for every *b*, 10 for
every *c*, and 20 for every *d*.

    Total: _____

If you have a score of 60 or less, chances are your lifestyle and activity level contribute to your difficulty in losing weight or maintaining your weight loss. Turn to page 330 to learn more about how normal daily activity can contribute to your effort to control your weight.

## Exercise:

82. Mark each statement that is true for you: _____

    a. I walk at least 30 minutes a day most days of the week.

    b. I use a pedometer and frequently reach 10,000 steps each day.

    c. I ride my bicycle several times a week.

    d. I know how to swim and there is a pool near me that I use regularly.

    e. There are exercise classes near me that I enjoy several times a week.

    f. I play tennis or golf regularly.

    g. I play other competitive sports regularly.

    h. I frequently participate in the martial arts such as Tai Chi or Tai Kwan Do.

    i. It is important to me to be active almost every day.

    j. I have a workout video/DVD that I use several times a week.

    k. I have two or three enjoyable physical activities that keep me active most days of the year.

    l. I lift weights several times each week.

If you weren't able to mark any of these statements, don't despair. You've got plenty of company: 60 percent of Americans describe themselves as sedentary. On the other hand, exercise is an important aspect of a healthy lifestyle and of managing your weight. For most people, exercise makes long-term weight loss and maintenance easier, and it makes you feel good. Turn to page 354 for help in figuring out how you can integrate exercise into your life.

If you marked 1 or 2 of these statements true—good for you. You are well on your way to having an active life that will make losing weight and maintaining that weight loss easier. You can turn to page 354 as well to find out how to make exercise a regular part of your life.

If you marked 3 or more of these statements, then congratulations; chances are you are exercising regularly. And you have enough variety to keep you interested, healthy, and injury free. Good for you.

83. Mark each statement that is true for you:

   a. I have so many responsibilities that I don't have time for myself.

   b. I don't have any friends who exercise.

   c. Most people I know are overweight.

   d. I am too busy to exercise.

   e. I don't enjoy exercise.

   f. There is no place for me to exercise.

   g. I don't know how to exercise.

   h. I'm uncomfortable in a gym because of how I look.

   i. I have never been in good shape.

   j. I have never exercised regularly.

   k. I feel silly when I exercise.

   l. I feel incompetent when I exercise.

Give yourself 1 point for each of the statements you marked as true for you. If you scored 5 points or more, you have some serious resistance to exercise. For help figuring out how to get past these problems, check out page 355.

If you scored between 3 and 5, you have good attitudes about exercise but probably need to increase the frequency. This may be a time issue or this may be a pleasure issue. To learn about how you might be able to address these problems, turn to page 355.

If you scored 2 or less, then congratulations! You have a good attitude about exercise and you do it regularly.

# THE ANSWER KEY

Use these pages to keep track of your answers so you can tally them up.

## PART 1: FOOD PREFERENCES

### 1. Are you a Carnimore? _____

Count carbs _____
Count cals _____
Count fat _____

### 2. Are you a Milk Mavin? _____

Count carbs _____
Count cals _____
Count fat _____

### 3. Are you a VegeCarian? _____

Count carbs _____
Count cals _____
Count fat _____

### 4. Are you a Starch Stealer? _____

Count carbs _____
Count cals _____
Count fat _____

### 5. Are you a Sweets Eater? _____

Count carbs _____
Count cals _____
Count fat _____

### 6. Are you a Junk-Food Junkie? _____

Count carbs _____
Count cals _____
Count fat _____

### 7. Are you a Waterless Wonder? _____

Count carbs _____
Count cals _____
Count fat _____

### 8–15. Are you a PROP taster? _____

Count carbs _____
Count cals _____
Count fat _____

## PART 2: DIETING HISTORY

### 16–22. What makes you feel full? _____

Count carbs _____
Count cals _____
Count fat _____

### 23–30. Has dieting affected the way you eat? _____

_____

_____

_____

### 31–36. Do you have, or are you at risk for, an eating disorder? _____

_____

## PART 3: MEDICAL HISTORY

### 37. Your own history: ___

Count carbs _____
Count cals _____
Count fat _____

### 38. Your family history: ___

Count carbs _____
Count cals _____
Count fat _____

**39. Do you have metabolic syndrome?** ____

Count carbs _____
Count cals _____
Count fat _____

## PART 4: FAMILY HERITAGE

**40–42. Does your genetic makeup play a role in your weight?** _____

_____

**43–47. Do your experiences growing up play a role in your weight?** ___

_____

## PART 5: HOW YOU EAT

**48–55. Do your eating habits play a role in your weight?** _____

_____

**56–63. Do you eat to address a non-hunger need?** _____

_____

## PART 6: LIFESTYLE

**64–72. Does eating out contribute to your weight?** _____

Count carbs _____
Count cals _____
Count fat _____

**73–81. Does your activity level contribute to your weight?** _____

_____

**82. Do you need to excercise more frequently?** _____

_____

**83. Do you have a resistance to exercise?** _____

_____

# SCORING THE QUESTIONNAIRE

Now is the time when we tally up all the diet preferences and see which one is right for you.

Count up all the points you put in the Counting Carbohydrates, Counting Calories, and Counting Fats categories.

Counting Carbs: _____

Counting Cals: _____

Counting Fats: _____

The maximum number of points you could get in any single diet is 16 (it is even lower if you skipped the first seven questions). The diet that gets the most points is the diet for you. You should go to the chapter on that type of diet and read up on it. For example, if you scored highest in the Counting Fats category, then turn to chapter 8 and read up on the whys and wherefores of counting fats. If instead you scored most in the Counting Carbs category, then turn to chapter 6.

Each diet chapter starts with the big picture of the diet—what you should be eating and why. There is also a list of foods in serving sizes that are calculated in the scale that is appropriate for your diet. For example, the Counting Carbs plan has a list of foods in quantities that have less than 5 grams of carbohydrates. Lastly, you will find a 7-day eating plan to give you some guidance in how to put these foods together to make an actual diet. These are diets that I developed based on the research I have done in nutrition.

But what if you ended up evenly split between two diet varieties? There is a maximum of 16 points, and it's possible for someone to score 5 and 5 and 5 and be completely confused. In that case, you should go one extra step: The first section, questions 1–15, are the questions that look at food preferences. Which plan gets the highest score there? (If there was a tie, count both.)

Food Preferences score:

Counting Carbs: _____

Counting Cals: _____

Counting Fats: _____

Next, look at questions 16–30 in the Dieting History section, and write down which plan gets the highest score there. (Again, if there was a tie, count both.)

Dieting History score:

Counting Carbs: _____

Counting Cals: _____

Counting Fats: _____

Third, look at questions 37 and 38 in the Medical History section, and write down which plan gets the highest score there. (If there was a tie, count both.)

Medical History score:

Counting Carbs: _____

Counting Cals: _____

Counting Fats: _____

Then, look at the section on metabolic syndrome, question 39, and write down which plan gets the highest score there.

Metabolic Syndrome score:

Counting Carbs: _____

Counting Cals: _____

Counting Fats: _____

Finally, look at the section on Eating Out, questions 64–72, and mark which plan gets the highest score there.

Eating Out score:

Counting Carbs: _____

Counting Cals: _____

Counting Fats: _____

Whichever one of those gets the majority of these points is the plan most likely to fit you perfectly. But, before you continue, you should recognize that the fact that you may have scored highly on two diets suggests that both have qualities that will appeal to you. Consider reading up on both diets to see which aspects of each one will fit you best. Now let's go on to part 3.

PART

# THE PERFECT FIT
# BASIC DIETS

NOW THAT YOU'VE KEPT a 4-day eating and exercise diary and finished your questionnaire, you know a lot more about what, how, and why you enjoy certain foods. And you've probably figured out which of the three basic diets is the best fit for you: the Counting Carbohydrates Diet, the Counting Calories Diet, or the Counting Fats Diet.

In part 3, I'll walk you through each basic diet and explain:

- Why it's likely to be the best weight-loss strategy for you

- The essential principles of the diet as well as what the most up-to-date research has to say about why and how you'll lose weight on this diet

- How to make this kind of diet work for you so you can reach and maintain your desired weight

At the end of each chapter, I'll also give you a list of foods that are allowed on each diet and offer you a weeklong meal plan that can be modified from week to week.

You need to read only the chapter about the basic diet you've been paired with, but if you're still not sure which diet is the best fit for you, then you may want to read about all three of them.

I have created versions of these three basic diet plans based on my research in nutrition and experiences with my own patients. They're similar to other diets in the same category but with unique twists to make them the most effective, the most easily maintained, and the safest version of each diet. Essentially, each of them emphasizes foods that are as fresh and unprocessed as possible with a low–saturated fat content and a low glycemic load. (If any of these terms are unfamiliar to you now, trust me, they won't be by the time you're done selecting and customizing your diet.)

In part 4, I'll show you how to tailor your basic diet to fit your food preferences, medical history, and lifestyle to a T. But right now, my job is to give you a chance to familiarize yourself with how your basic diet will work to help you find and maintain your desired weight.

# CHAPTER 6

# THE COUNTING CARBOHYDRATES DIET

I T HAS BEEN HAILED as a "diet revolution," but it's really been more like the world's oldest food fight. The low-carbohydrate diet has been around for more than 2,000 years; the ancient Greek athletes ate a diet consisting exclusively of meat while preparing for the Olympics. But the diet got its most recent start in 1972 with the publication of *Dr. Atkins' Diet Revolution* by Manhattan-based cardiologist Robert Atkins, M.D. That book and its incredible success triggered a true revolution in diet strategy. Along with Atkins have come a slew of other low-carb diets: the Scarsdale diet, the Zone diet, Sugar Busters, Protein Power, Suzanne Somers's *Get Skinny on Fabulous Food*, and, most recently, the South Beach diet. All maintain that the reason we are fat—and getting fatter—is that we eat too many carbohydrates, and carbs make us that way.

Traditional medicine has recoiled in horror at the notion of a diet heavy on meats (and fat) and skimpy on fruits, vegetables, and breads. It seemed clear that such a diet would be unhealthy and increase the risk of heart disease and other health problems. The truth is that although this diet runs counter to many of the ideas cherished by generations of doctors, recent studies show that it is a safe and effective choice for many dieters.

In this chapter we will look first at who does well on this diet. Then I'll walk you through the basic principles of a low-carbohydrate diet. If you have a grip on how this diet works, you will be able to make it work better for you. We'll briefly review what we know, and don't know, about its safety. The Perfect Fit Counting Carbohydrates Diet is described in detail in the next section, followed by a list of no- and low-carbohydrate foods and a 7-day eating plan. At the end of the chapter, you'll find some recipes that will help you stay within the guidelines of this diet.

There are aspects of this diet that definitely make losing weight easier for some folks. First of all, you will be eating very filling and satisfying foods. And you will be avoiding many of the foods that seem to be easy to overeat, such as bread, chips, and sweets. However, on this diet, you will never feel deprived. While your choice of foods in this diet is the most limited of all the diets, the foods you are allowed to eat are some of the richest, most luxurious foods available.

*The Perfect Fit for June (lost 28 pounds)*
*I'm 36 years old and I'm finally at a weight that's right for me. I was never heavy until I got into my twenties. That's when my marriage started going bad, and the pounds just appeared. Now I know I'm a stress eater, but back then I couldn't figure out where the pounds were coming from. I just knew I wasn't happy—not with my marriage, not with my body.*

*The first diet I ever tried was Slim Fast. I followed the directions and drank two cans of the drink—one in the morning and one in the afternoon and then I'd try to eat a sensible dinner. That was hard. I was starving by the time I sat down to eat what was my first real meal of the day—at 6:00 P.M. But I lost 10 pounds and felt pretty good. But, of course, the weight came back right away—with a whole bunch more.*

*After that I tried a lot of different things: I tried these pills that you took right before a meal with a whole bunch of water. I lost 14 pounds in 2 weeks but it seems like it came back just about overnight once I'd finished the pills. I tried a low-fat diet and I lost 20 pounds on that. But I couldn't eat like that. I just couldn't keep it up and I was hungry all the time. I was eating huge portions, but I was still hungry.*

*I swear I tried just about every diet that was ever created. None of them felt really right. Oh, I might be able to stick with it for a few weeks, but then I'd get bored with what I was "allowed" to eat and then it would be over. I'd slip back into my old ways and just give up—at least for a while.*

*I remember the first time I tried a low-carb diet. It was a long time ago when they first got real popular around here and it seems like everyone was on it, so I tried it. It tasted good, but it made me feel bad. Like I was filled with grease. So when the questionnaire pushed me toward a low-carb diet I was disappointed. Been there, tried that. But I'd tried just about everything else, too, so I tried it again.*

*This low-carb diet steered me away from fatty foods and more toward lean meats and there were plenty of vegetables in it and even some sweets. And I felt good—great, really. And I lost weight. In the first week, I lost 5 pounds. I knew that it was water weight, but it showed up on the scale and that made me feel good right away. And the weight loss continued: I went from 200 to 172 in just a few months. It was easy to stick to and I was never hungry. I liked the foods and I liked the way I felt. I thought I really had found the perfect diet for me.*

*After a few months, though, I noticed that I was craving things that I wasn't "supposed" to eat. So I went back to the book. I knew I was supposed to add more carbs, but hadn't wanted to do it because I was doing so well on the very low-carb part. I realized I'd probably maxed out what I could do eating that way. If I was going to stick with it, I really needed more variety in my diet. So I started adding some of the carbs back. Just the stuff I really wanted. And I paid attention to how it made me feel.*

*One thing I noticed right away was that eating pasta made me feel really tired. I don't like how that feels so I still don't eat much pasta. I loved having the fruit back in my diet. I love sweets and the fruit provides me with that taste so that I don't crave other stuff so much.*

*The questionnaire also showed me I was a stress eater. I saw that I craved carbs the most when I was upset. Knowing that has made it a lot easier to deal with. And I realized that I didn't have to have a cookie when I'm stressed because that feeling goes away whether I eat something or not. And that was a great thing to realize.*

*I'm pretty happy with my weight now, And though maybe I'll always think, maybe 5 more pounds, I'm at my goal. I gave away all my fat clothes and I have a new wardrobe and I think I look pretty darned good. One of the great benefits of losing this weight was that some of my friends and my family saw that I could do it, so they've tried to find their perfect diet, too. Everyone is getting involved and it's a good feeling seeing everyone getting better. It feels good to be a role model. I feel like I showed them it could be done and now they are doing it for themselves. Because they know they can. I like the way I eat now. I really do. And I know that I'll never go back to the way I used to eat. Because I've found the way to eat that's right for me.*

## WHO DOES WELL ON A CARB-COUNTING DIET?

If the questionnaire directed you here, the answer to that question is probably you. What aspects of eating make a good carb counter? First, you have to like the food. If you can't imagine a meal without meat or a life without cheese, you've come to the right place. If a life where muffins and pasta are the occasional treat rather than daily fare appeals, step right up. If you would rather have a taste of a really wonderful rich food, rather than a big bowl of pasta, come on in.

It's not just the food. Health factors may also contribute to the success of the carb counter. If you have high triglycerides and a low HDL cholesterol then a carb-counting diet may be just right for you. If diabetes runs in your family, if you carry your weight around your middle, this may be the diet to deflate that spare tire and make you thinner and healthier. Lifestyle is important: If you can't snack or prefer just the three squares a day, this is a good diet for you. If you eat out or travel regularly, this may do the trick. All these factors were touched on by the questionnaire and your answers led you here. Come on in.

## THE BASICS OF A LOW-CARBOHYDRATE DIET

**Do carbs make you fat?** You might assume that if getting rid of carbs makes you lose weight, then it is carbohydrates that made you fat in the first place. And you might be right. Not all carbohydrates and not everyone, but it is clear that some carbohydrates will make some individuals gain weight. I give more details on this in part 4 but let me give you the basics here.

**So which carbohydrates?** One thing you may not know about carbohydrates is that they are all broken down into sugar once they are in your system. It's true for sweets, it's true for bread and pasta, it's true for fruits and vegetables. The big difference between these foods is how fast they make this change, and how much sugar they turn into. Some carbs are broken down very rapidly by your body, and what that means is that a big load of sugar is sent into your bloodstream over a very short period of time.

Your body will respond to this sugar load by releasing a big dose of insulin—and that's where the trouble starts. Insulin's main job in the body is to help the cells of your body take up the sugar being provided to them in the foods you eat. The sugar is important because it is the fuel that makes your body work, and the insulin is essential because without it the fuel doesn't get to the tiny engines that do the work of living and breathing. But, in your body, as in comedy, timing is everything. Sending a gusher of sugar into your system means that your body has to respond with a big load of insulin. And that big surge of insulin is what causes the problem.

You see, insulin affects many parts of the body—and many of those effects you just don't want any part of. First, insulin makes your body a fat-storage machine. The high insulin levels tell your body that this is a time of plenty and that you should be storing away fat for hard times that may be coming later. This response was useful in the prehistoric plains of early hominids, but it's

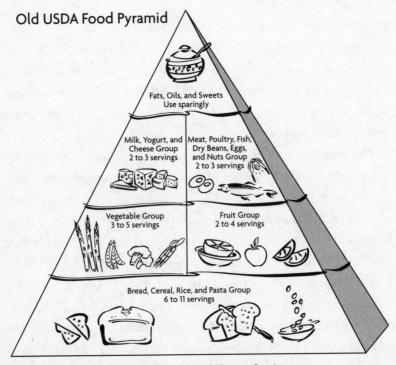

Old USDA Food Pyramid

Fats, Oils, and Sweets
Use sparingly

Milk, Yogurt, and Cheese Group
2 to 3 servings

Meat, Poultry, Fish, Dry Beans, Eggs, and Nuts Group
2 to 3 servings

Vegetable Group
3 to 5 servings

Fruit Group
2 to 4 servings

Bread, Cereal, Rice, and Pasta Group
6 to 11 servings

© USDA and U.S. Department of Health and Human Services

much less helpful in the well-stocked world of today, where obesity has replaced starvation as the number one nutritional problem in the world. Elevated insulin levels also drive your blood pressure up; it promotes atherosclerosis or hardening of the arteries; it can mess up your cholesterol. Chronically high insulin promotes heart disease.

So some carbohydrates do end up making you fat and unhealthy. Some, but not all. So how can you tell the difference? It's all in the timing. When carbs are transformed into sugar slowly, only small amounts of insulin are needed at any one moment and you don't go into a fat-storage mode. The carbohydrates that make you fat are those that are broken down quickly. You want slow carbs. Most carbs start off slow, but thanks to our modern food-processing miracles many slow carbs have been turned into fast carbs by the

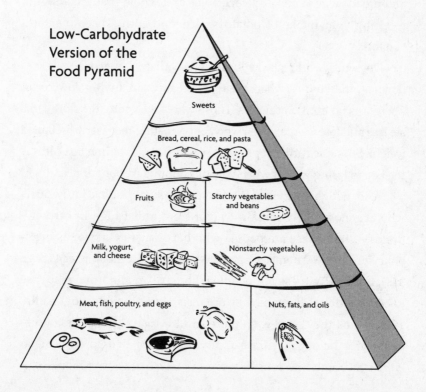

Low-Carbohydrate Version of the Food Pyramid

Sweets

Bread, cereal, rice, and pasta

Fruits

Starchy vegetables and beans

Milk, yogurt, and cheese

Nonstarchy vegetables

Meat, fish, poultry, and eggs

Nuts, fats, and oils

time we buy them in the store. Whole grains are slow carbs; it takes time to break them down to their sugary components. But if a machine grinds them into tiny particles that are easy to digest, you've taken a slow carb and made it into a fast carb. Highly refined carbs are quickly broken down by your body and require high levels of insulin, and that promotes weight gain.

There are some foods that naturally stimulate high levels of insulin. These are white potatoes, rice, corn—in short, starches. Eating these foods can send your insulin up as easily as if you were eating plain sugar. In part 4 I give you some details on how to tell slow carbs from fast carbs using what is known as the glycemic load of a food. The short version is that if you are trying to avoid carbohydrates, you don't have to get rid of them all. Just get rid of the ones that send your insulin to the stratosphere. That means replacing highly processed foods like baked goods (cookies, cakes, chips, and bread) with fruits and vegetables and whole-grain foods. And reducing your intake of potatoes, rice, and corn. That's the short version.

Does this work? David Ludwig, a pediatrician at Harvard, has done several studies where he replaced fast carbs with slow carbs. There was no limit on calories. Those who were eating the slow carbs ate less and lost weight; those who kept on eating the fast carbs gained weight. So, some carbs do promote weight gain. Avoiding fast carbs is the key to losing weight when you are counting carbohydrates.

**And which individuals?** There are clearly some individuals who are more likely to gain weight from a diet high in carbohydrates. Who? These are people who have what is known as metabolic syndrome. There are details on this syndrome in part 4 (page 317), but briefly these are people who have an abnormal response to carbohydrates because they are resistant to the effect of insulin. That means they need even more insulin than other people do to deal with the sugar from carbohydrates. For people with metabolic syndrome, the consumption of fast carbs is even more damaging, because they have even more insulin floating around in their bodies.

This is not some tiny fraction of the population. One in five Americans has metabolic syndrome. And most of them don't even know they have it. If you have metabolic syndrome (and you will know after you take the questionnaire), you should avoid fast carbohydrates no matter which diet you end up on.

**How does a low-carbohydrate diet work?** In a low-carbohydrate diet you won't just limit your carbohydrates to slow carb, although that is certainly part of it. You will eat fewer carbohydrates overall and you will get most of your calories from proteins and fats. Hearing this you might wonder (as many doctors and nutritionists have) how this change will cause weight loss. Pound for pound, fat contains more calories than carbohydrates and proteins contain the same number of calories. How can eating more of these help you lose weight?

First of all, despite the sales rap, a successful low-carbohydrate diet is a low-calorie diet. The carbohydrates it prohibits are the most abundant foods in the American diet; up to 60 percent of our calories each day come from carbs. Eliminate them, and chances are you will be taking in far fewer calories, even if you eat more of the foods you're allowed.

Let me take a second to compare the low-carb diet to its opposite: the low-fat diet. On the surface the two diets couldn't be more different. A low-carb diet has you eating lots of protein and fat. A low-fat diet wants you to eat lots of carbs and much less fat. But both the low-fat and low-carbohydrate diets share one important characteristic: The foods prohibited on both these diets are some of the most fattening foods in the marketplace. Which foods? The high-fat, high-carbohydrate foods that have taken an increasingly large role in our diets: chips, cookies, donuts, and pastries. While coming at these foods from opposite directions, both diets eliminate many of the same calorie-rich, nutrition-poor foods.

Moreover, the foods remaining in the low-carb diet, proteins

## GLYCEMIC LOAD

You may not have heard of glycemic load, but maybe you have heard of the glycemic index. What's the difference? The glycemic index tells you how quickly a particular carbohydrate turns into sugar. It doesn't tell you how much of that carbohydrate is in a serving of that particular food. You need to know both things to understand a food's effect on blood sugar. That is where glycemic load comes in. For example, the carbohydrate found in a carrot breaks down very rapidly into sugar, so it has a high glycemic index. There isn't a lot of that carbohydrate in a serving of carrots, however, so it has a low glycemic load. Glycemic load gives you a better sense of how carbohydrates actually work in the diet. Here is a short list of some common foods and their glycemic loads.

| Food | Glycemic Load | Food | Glycemic Load |
|---|---|---|---|
| Apple | 6 | Jell-O, sugar-free | 0 |
| Avocado | 0 | Honey | 10 |
| Bacon | 0 | Lettuce (all varieties) | 0 |
| Bagel, plain | 25 | Mango | 8 |
| Banana | 12 | Milk | 4 |
| Beef | 0 | Oatmeal, plain | 0 |
| Bread, seven-grain | 8 | Olive oil | 0 |
| Bread, white | 10 | Orange | 5 |
| Butter | 0 | Potato | 26 |
| Carrot | 3 | Raisin bran | 12 |
| Cheese | 0 | Rice, white | 14 |
| Chicken | 0 | Sour cream | 8 |
| Chickpeas | 8 | Soy milk | 8 |
| Couscous, cooked | 23 | Strawberry | 1 |
| Cucumber | 0 | Sugar | 7 |
| Egg | 0 | Yogurt, low-fat, fruit-flavored | 10 |
| English muffin | 11 | | |

and fats and slow carbs are some of the most filling foods we eat. While it's possible—even easy—to consume loads of potato chips, overeating high-protein, high-fat foods like steak or creamy sauces is more difficult. They make you too full. Sure, we do it every Thanksgiving, but the overstuffed feeling we get afterward is enough to remind us not to do it again—at least not for another year. So a low-carb diet makes you feel fuller and you eat less.

Hard to believe? But it's true. In studies comparing people on a diet that restricts carbohydrates to those on a low-fat, calorie-restricted diet, the low-carb group took in just as few calories as those on the calorie-restricted diet eating low-fat foods, even though the low carbers weren't counting calories. They ate fewer calories without even trying.

Finally, there is the almost instant weight loss seen in the low-carb diet. One of the first dieters to promote the low-carb diet, eighteenth-century coffin maker William Banting, spoke glowingly of the immediate results he saw. "The great charms and comfort of the system," he noted in a now famous letter, "are that its effects are palpable within a week of trial and creates a natural stimulus to persevere for a few weeks more." The diet helped him lose 46 of his 202 pounds in the course of a year, at the age of 66.

Traditionally, doctors have scoffed at this claim—not because it isn't true. Even the most hard-core critics acknowledge the fact that low-carbohydrate dieters can lose several pounds in the first few days of this diet. Why? Because by eating a diet with virtually no carbohydrates in it, low-carb dieters get rid of the sugar stored in the liver (glycogen) within the first 2 to 3 days of the diet, and each pound of sugar comes attached to 1½ pounds of water. On average, we store between 1 and 2 pounds of sugar in our livers. Cut out the carbs, and—poof!—5 pounds of sugar and water will virtually melt away.

Doctors who scoff at this say that this isn't true weight loss. You're not losing fat, just water. And the water weight will come back as soon as you reintroduce carbohydrates. Nevertheless, that early, almost effortless weight loss provides encouragement when dieters first start this eating plan, and many dieters find this useful.

## A WORD ON SAFETY

Doctors have been concerned about the safety of this diet for hundreds of years. The criticism of recent generations of doctors has been that a diet so high in fat will increase your risk of heart disease by increasing cholesterol.

That doesn't happen. Several recent studies have examined this issue, and it turns out that while LDL (bad) cholesterol stays about the same, HDL (good) cholesterol increases—and that reduces your risk of heart disease. And triglycerides, which increase risk of heart disease, decrease dramatically on this diet. In my own research, we looked at more than five hundred diets and compared the safety and effectiveness of low-carbohydrate diets with diets that restricted fats or calories. We were particularly interested in the effects of a low-carb diet on cholesterol. We found that on average those on low-carb diets had no change in their total cholesterol. So, while many doctors remain suspicious of this diet, the research suggests that for most people this diet is safe.

## THE PERFECT FIT COUNTING CARBOHYDRATES BASIC DIET

So what does the Counting Carbohydrates Diet look like? First, it is a two-part program. In the first phase, carbohydrates are dramatically restricted. This type of limitation helps dieters lose weight immediately and continue to lose weight as long as they maintain the diet. But the sheer monotony of this diet—clearly a factor in making the diet so effective initially—also makes it virtually impossible to maintain for the long run. So, just when you are thinking that you just couldn't face another day of cheese omelets, salmon steaks, and salad, the diet adds back many of the carbohydrates you crave.

With the addition of these foods, you will be able to continue to lose weight until you reach your target. Moreover, this is a diet you will be able to continue to enjoy, a satisfying eating program that will help you maintain your target weight, not just for now but for life.

## STARTING THE COUNTING CARBOHYDRATES DIET

In this initial phase of the Counting Carbohydrates Diet, you will be restricted to a diet containing around 30 grams of carbohydrates per day. This means that the only carbohydrates you'll be able to eat are one or two servings of dairy products and green vegetables. There will be no breads, no pastries, no pastas, a very limited amount of fruits, and no sweets. On the other hand, you will be able to eat your fill of seafood, meat, poultry, eggs, and cheese, and many (though not all) vegetables.

Restricting your body's intake of carbohydrates to this extent will shift the way your body uses food for energy. In the diet you eat now, most of the food you take in is converted to sugar (glucose), and that sugar is the fuel used to power all the body's functions. When you start on the Counting Carbohydrates Diet and limit your carbs to 30 grams per day, you will not be eating enough sugar to run your body, so your body will switch over to its back-up fuel—fat. Your body will convert the food you eat, not to sugar, but to microscopic portions of fat, known as ketone bodies.

After several days on this diet, you'll notice many things: First, you will see an immediate change in your weight. This is the water you lose as you burn up the sugar stored in your liver. (Average weight loss will be 3 to 5 pounds.) You may find that you make a few extra trips to the bathroom as you lose this excess water, but that should last only a couple of days. And you may notice a slightly sweet taste in your mouth. That sweet taste is a by-product of the ketone bodies, and it proves that your body has switched over to this alternative fuel.

But I don't want you to depend on that sweet taste to tell you when your body is burning fats rather than sugar. It's not reliable enough. While you are on this initial phase of the diet, I want you to check your urine for the presence of those little fat bodies. If you go to just about any drugstore, you can ask for strips to check your urine for ketones. You'll get a bottle filled with little strips of (usually) white paper. When you dip these strips into your urine, they will turn pink (sometimes purple or other colors; check the label) and that will tell you if you have really gotten rid of enough of the carbohydrates to force your body to burn fats rather than sugar. I call this being "in the pink."

The main reason to check your urine daily is to make sure that you are following the diet as closely as possible. But there is an additional benefit: These ketones will help curb your appetite, and that is important, especially in the early stages of a new way of eating, until you learn how to eat less and be satisfied. Portion size is, to a very large extent, learned based on portions that have satisfied you in the past. Part of any eating plan is to help you relearn a new and healthful portion size and get away from the supersize insanity that has swept the nation.

In addition to checking your urine every day while on this diet, I want you to take a multivitamin every day, if you don't already. All calorie-restricted diets—not just this one—run the risk of allowing you to leave out some of the aspects of a proper diet. One vitamin a day. It's not hard and, although you may not need it, it won't hurt. I put all my patients on multivitamins. I mean, what's the downside? It doesn't really matter which multivitamin you take. Women should take vitamins with iron, plus calcium supplements. If you are post-

## GETTING "IN THE PINK"

Sometimes it takes several days before you get "in the pink." If it takes longer than that, chances are you are still taking in too many carbohydrates. There are two possibilities here: First, carbohydrates are sneaking into your diet without you knowing it. This can happen very easily, so check the carbohydrate content of everything you are eating and drinking to look for hidden carbs.

Alternatively, you may be taking in only 30 grams of carbohydrates per day, but your body needs even less to make this switch. If that is the case, I would recommend eliminating all carbohydrates from your diet (including the milk in your coffee), at which point the strips will turn the proper color; you can then add back carbs a little at a time and see at what level you start to lose that color. That will become your level of carbohydrate restriction. Once you achieve this state of fat burning—once you are "in the pink"—you need to check your urine every day to make sure you stay there. Carbohydrates are ubiquitous, and it's very easy for them to find their way back onto your plate. Checking your urine every morning allows you to know that you are limiting your carbohydrates enough to lose weight. When you start to lose that color, you need to think, What did I eat today or yesterday that could be increasing my carbohydrate load?

menopausal, you can skip the iron; check with your doctor if you have any questions about whether you need it. For men, just the basic multivitamin should do the trick.

One last thing on this diet: Make sure you drink enough water. That's eight 8-ounce glasses per day—64 ounces of fluid—day in, day out. And coffee and alcohol don't count when you're figuring up how much you drink. One simple rule of thumb: Your urine should look very much like water. If it's dark or yellow, you aren't drinking enough.

Getting enough fluid is important no matter what you are eating, but it takes on special importance with this diet. Why? Well, first of all you will be eating less of the kinds of foods that contain a lot of water. Carbohydrates contain lots of water—much more than proteins or fats. Plus, proteins in particular can increase the workload on your kidneys. You need to have enough water to flush the wastes from proteins through. Finally, ketones act as diuretics; they make you urinate more. You need to drink enough to keep up with what you put out.

I have included a list of no- and low-carbohydrate foods in this chapter as well as a 7-day eating plan for the early Counting Carbohydrates Diet to give you some idea of how you can eat with this type of restriction. Basically, you will be eating eggs, cheese, seafood, meat, and green vegetables. All are important components of the diet. Because of the nature of this diet, you will be eating a relatively high level of fat. But it will be primarily mono- and polyunsaturated fats (the "good" fats) and relatively low in saturated fats (the "bad" fats).

Multiple studies have shown that, in general, low-carbohydrate dieters are able to eat this type of diet without adversely affecting their own cholesterol profile. If you are concerned about your cholesterol, however, or have a history of high LDL (bad) cholesterol, I recommend that you talk to your doctor before you start this diet and get your cholesterol rechecked after you have been on the diet for 3 to 6 months to make sure that your cholesterol is moving in the right direction.

While you can eat as much of the fats and proteins that contain no carbs as you like, everything containing carbohydrates should be measured and weighed for the first couple of weeks at least and periodically thereafter. Carbohydrates are easy to overeat, and measuring them is a good reality check on what your true carbohydrate intake is.

Exactly how long you need to stay on this very restrictive phase of the diet is up to you. Between 1 and 3 months is what I generally recommend. Less than 1 month, and you cheat yourself out of the benefits of this type of diet by bailing out too soon. On the other hand, most people stop losing weight (as quickly) after 3 months, usually because they can't stick to this monotonous diet any longer.

My recommendation is to follow the 30-gram Counting Carbohydrates Diet for 2 to 3 months. If you find yourself wanting to cheat (or actually cheating), then you have to consider increasing your carbohydrate content in order to give yourself some of the variety you are craving. Even though people on this diet do not value lots of variety in their diets, you are programmed at the genetic level to want some, so chances are you will. My patients certainly do.

## MAINTAINING THE COUNTING CARBOHYDRATES DIET

By the time you get to this phase of the diet, you will be well on your way to your target weight. In this second phase of the Counting Carbohydrates Diet, you will be able to eat up to 100 grams of carbohydrates per day. This is still a very limited carbohydrate diet. At the most, you will be getting about a third of your calories from carbohydrates. That's about half of what the average American diet usually provides.

But, as you probably know by now, not all carbohydrates are created equal, and so the carbohydrates you will be adding back into your diet will be limited to fruits and vegetables, with occasional whole-grain pastas and breads. These carbohydrates have a low or moderate glycemic load. You will not be adding back sweets, chips, or baked goods. These high-glycemic-index carbohydrates are foods that provide too many carbohydrates and too many calories. Moreover, because they have a moderate to high glycemic load, they make you hungrier. These are foods that tantalize but can't satisfy. So, even in this phase of the diet, the only carbohydrates allowed are complex carbs, primarily those with a low glycemic load. Fats will make up almost half of the calories consumed, and proteins fill in the rest.

On the 100-gram Counting Carbohydrates Diet, there is no need to check your urine. Once you eat this many carbohydrates, you will go back to using sugar (glucose) as your primary fuel. You will still lose weight for the same reason you were losing weight on the earlier diet: You will be eating fewer calories, and you will be avoiding the types of foods that promote high levels of insulin, since insulin can promote fat storage over fat usage.

One word of advice before you get started on this diet: The theory behind it is that by severely restricting intake of carbohydrates—the food that makes up the majority of the calories most of us take in on a given day—we will end up consuming fewer calories. The greater satisfaction associated with eating a larger percentage of your calories from proteins and fats undoubtedly contributes to this decrease in appetite. But if you end up sneaking carbohydrates back into your diet, you will be undermining the ways in which it is designed to make you lose weight. You'll end up with the worst possible diet: one that's high in fats and proteins *and* refined carbohydrates. If you add back the refined carbohydrates, you are just eating more of everything, and that is a sure way to gain weight.

On the other hand, if you feel good on this diet, and if it allows you to achieve and maintain your desired weight, there is no reason to stop it once you have achieved your ideal weight. This diet is balanced enough to allow you to continue on it indefinitely.

Now, on to the foods and the diet!

# FOOD LIST FOR THE COUNTING CARBS BASIC DIET

## NO CARBOHYDRATE CONTENT

**MEAT, POULTRY, AND SEAFOOD** (Virtually all are carbohydrate-free—exceptions found in Very Low Carb Foods list on the following page.)

### FATS AND OILS

Almond oil

Avocado oil

Canola oil

Margarine

Olive oil

Sesame oil

Shortening

Soybean oil

Sunflower seed oil

### VEGETABLES

Arugula

Lettuce

Watercress

### CHEESE AND OTHER DAIRY PRODUCTS

Babybel cheese

Blue cheese

Bonbel cheese

Brie

Butter

Camembert cheese

Fontina cheese

Havarti cheese

Muenster cheese

### SPICES AND CONDIMENTS

Capers

Lemon juice

Mayonnaise

Mustard

Sugar substitutes

Vinegar

### BEVERAGES

Coffee

Seltzers (including most
  unsweetened flavored seltzers)

Soft drinks, diet

Soup, beef and chicken broth

Tea

Water (including unsweetened
  flavored varieties)

## SWEETS

| | |
|---|---|
| D-Zerta gelatin mix | Jell-O (sugar-free) |

**VERY LOW CARB FOODS** (This list provides you with the serving sizes that will give you about 5 grams of carbohydrates; these aren't the amounts you must eat, but they will give you an idea of how much carbohydrate is contained in these naturally low-carb foods.)

## MEAT, POULTRY, AND SEAFOOD

| | |
|---|---|
| Abalone | 3 oz |
| Caviar | 5 oz |
| Clams | 3 oz/5 clams |
| Eggs | 5 eggs |
| Frankfurters | 5 franks |
| Ham | 10 oz |
| Lobster | 2 cups |
| Luncheon meats | 2 slices |
| Mussels | 3 oz/1 cup |
| Oysters | 3 oz/6 cooked |
| Pâté | 4 oz |
| Roe | 6 oz |
| Sausage | 5 oz |
| Scallops | 6 oz/10 pieces |
| Squid, fried | 3 oz |

## NUTS AND SEEDS

| | |
|---|---|
| Almond butter | 2 tbsp |
| Almonds | 1 oz/23 nuts |
| Brazil nuts | 6–8 nuts |
| Hazelnuts | 1 oz/25 nuts |
| Macadamia nuts | 1 oz/10–12 nuts |
| Peanut butter | 2 tbsp |
| Peanuts | 1 oz/¼ cup |
| Pecans | 1 oz/20 halves |
| Pepitas | 1 oz/120 seeds |

| | |
|---|---|
| Pine nuts | 1 oz/¼ cup |
| Pistachio nuts | 1 oz/¼ cup/about 47 nuts |
| Sunflower seeds | 1 oz |
| Walnuts | 1 oz/¼ cup |

## FRUITS AND VEGETABLES

| | |
|---|---|
| Apricot | 1 medium fruit |
| Artichoke hearts | 3 oz/4 pieces |
| Asparagus | 10 medium spears/½ cup cut |
| Avocado | 1 medium/1 cup |
| Bamboo shoots | ½ cup |
| Blueberries, fresh | ¼ cup/25 berries |
| Beans, green | ½ cup |
| Beans, mung, sprouted | 1 cup |
| Beans, Shelly | ½ cup |
| Beans, wax | ½ cup |
| Bean sprouts | 2 cups |
| Bok choy | 1 cup |
| Broccoli florets | 2 cups |
| Cabbage | 1 cup |
| Cauliflower | ⅕ head/1 cup florets |
| Celery | 1 cup/5 large ribs |
| Coleslaw | ½ cup |
| Collard greens | ½ cup |
| Cucumber | 2 cups |
| Eggplant | ⅔ cup cubed |
| Endive, raw | 2 cups |
| Hearts of palm | ⅔ cup |
| Kale | ⅔ cup |
| Mulberries, fresh | ⅓ cup/50 berries |
| Mushrooms | 5 oz/½ cup |
| Mustard greens | 2 cups |
| Okra | ½ cup |
| Olives | 15 |
| Peppers, green bell | 1 medium |

| | |
|---|---|
| Pickles, dill | 5 oz |
| Pickles, sweet | 1 oz |
| Radicchio | 1 cup |
| Radishes | 5 cups |
| Raspberries, fresh | 25 berries |
| Sauerkraut | ½ cup |
| Scallions | 1 cup |
| Shallots | 1 oz |
| Snow peas | ½ cup/15 pods |
| Spinach | 5 cups |
| Squash, spaghetti | ½ cup |
| Squash, yellow | 1 cup |
| Squash, zucchini | 1 cup |
| Strawberries | ½ cup |
| Swiss chard | 1 cup |
| Tomato, canned | ½ cup |
| Tomato, fresh | ⅔ cup/1 whole |
| Turnip greens, cooked | ½ cup |

## DAIRY

| | |
|---|---|
| Cool Whip | 5 tbsp |
| Cream, half-and-half | ½ cup |
| Egg substitute | 2 cups |
| Milk, whole or low-fat | ½ cup |
| Sour cream | ½ cup |
| Yogurt, plain | ⅓ cup |

## CHEESE

| | |
|---|---|
| American | 5 oz/5 slices |
| American, low-fat | 5 oz/5 slices |
| Bel Paese | 5 oz |
| Cheddar | 5 oz |
| Colby | 5 oz |
| Cottage cheese | ½ cup |
| Cream cheese | ⅔ cup/two 3-oz packages |

| | |
|---|---|
| Edam | 5 oz |
| Farmer cheese | 5 oz/½ cup |
| Feta | 5 oz |
| Gouda | 5 oz |
| Jarlsberg | 5 oz |
| Monterey Jack | 5 oz |
| Mozzarella | 5 oz |
| Neufchâtel | 5 oz |
| Parmesan | 5 oz |
| Provolone | 5 oz |
| Ricotta | 5 oz/½ cup |
| Romano | 5 oz |
| String cheese | 5 oz |
| Velveeta | 2 oz |

## CONDIMENTS

| | |
|---|---|
| Fruit spread | 1 tsp |
| Gravy (most canned and mix varieties) | ¼ cup |
| Horseradish | 4 oz |
| Ketchup | 1 tbsp/2 packets |
| Miso | 2 tbsp |
| Salad dressing (except low-fat) | 2 tbsp |
| Salsa | 5 oz/¼ cup |
| Sauces (most—some big exceptions, so check label) | 2 tbsp |
| Sesame butter (tahini) | 2 tbsp |
| Soup, onion | 1 cup |
| Tofu | ½ cup |

## DAILY MEAL PLANS
## FOR THE 30-GRAM COUNTING CARBS DIET

(Dishes in **bold print** are listed alphabetically in the recipe section at the end of the chapter on page 144.)

# DAY 1

### Breakfast

| | |
|---|---|
| 3-egg omelet (use only 1–2 yolks but all 3 whites) with ham and 2 ounces low-fat Cheddar cheese (cook in olive oil) | 3.5 g |
| Coffee with low-fat milk and sweetener (not sugar) | 1.5 g |

### A.M. Snack

| | |
|---|---|
| ½ cup cottage cheese with ½ cup cucumbers and radishes | 5.5 g |

### Lunch

| | |
|---|---|
| Chef's salad made with lettuce and spinach (total 4 cups), 1 ounce low-fat cheese, ham, 1 hard-boiled egg, and 4 artichoke hearts dressed with **Vinaigrette**. (If you use bottled salad dressing, check the carb content—should be 0.) | 4 g |

### P.M. Snack

| | |
|---|---|
| ½ avocado with **Vinaigrette** | 3 g |

### Dinner

| | |
|---|---|
| Chicken breast dredged in Parmesan cheese and sautéed in olive oil | 0 g |
| Broccoli florets with lemon juice | 3 g |
| ½ cup asparagus | 4 g |
| 2 cups raw spinach salad and ½ cup hearts of palm | 4 g |
| **Total carbohydrates for Day 1** | **28.5 g** |

# DAY 2

## Breakfast

| | |
|---|---:|
| 2 ounces smoked salmon and cream cheese | 1 g |
| 1 tomato, sliced | 6 g |
| Coffee with 1% milk and sweetener | 1.5 g |

## A.M. Snack

| | |
|---|---:|
| 10 radishes dipped in ranch dressing | 2 g |

## Lunch

| | |
|---|---:|
| **Cold Tomato Stuffed with Seafood** (try adding capers for a more sophisticated taste) | 6 g |

## P.M. Snack

| | |
|---|---:|
| 3 ham and low-fat cheese rolls (1 slice low-fat ham, 1 slice low-fat Swiss cheese, with a dab of mustard, rolled up) | 2 g |

## Dinner

| | |
|---|---:|
| 4 ounces broiled swordfish | 0 g |
| ½ cup sautéed mushrooms | 5 g |
| 2 cups arugula and lettuce salad with cucumbers and radishes topped with **Vinaigrette** | 1 g |
| D-Zerta gelatin topped with 2 tablespoons Cool Whip | 2 g |
| **Total carbohydrates for Day 2** | **26.5 g** |

# DAY 3

## Breakfast

| | |
|---|---:|
| Scrambled eggs (use 2 egg whites and 1 egg yolk) | 1.5 g |
| 2 slices Canadian bacon | 0 g |
| Coffee with 1% milk and sweetener | 1.5 g |

## A.M. Snack

| | |
|---|---:|
| 10–12 macadamia nuts | 4 g |

## Lunch

| | |
|---|---:|
| 4 cups Caesar salad (romaine lettuce, slivers of Parmesan cheese, no croutons, in Caesar dressing—check label for carb content) topped with 3 ounces broiled chicken breast | 4 g |

## P.M. Snack

| | |
|---|---:|
| Celery spread with 1 ounce cream cheese | 1 g |

## Dinner

| | |
|---|---:|
| Broiled or grilled lamb chop, served with sautéed mushrooms and onions | 5 g |
| 10 asparagus spears, steamed | 5 g |
| Broccoli florets, steamed | 3 g |
| Sugar-free Jell-O with 2 tablespoons Cool Whip | 2 g |
| **Total carbohydrates for Day 3** | **27 g** |

# DAY 4

## Breakfast

| | |
|---|---:|
| ½ cup low-fat plain yogurt | 8 g |
| ½ cup sliced strawberries | 5 g |
| 2 slices Canadian bacon | 0 g |
| Coffee with 1% milk and sweetener | 1.5 g |

## A.M. Snack

| | |
|---|---:|
| 1 ounce salmon spread with 1 tablespoon cream cheese | 1 g |

## Lunch

| | |
|---|---:|
| **Cold Tomato Stuffed with Seafood** | 6 g |
| 1 cup low-fat chicken consommé | 0 g |
| 5 green olives | 1 g |

### P.M. Snack

| 3 ham and low-fat cheese rolls | 2 g |
|---|---|

### Dinner

| Filet mignon, grilled or broiled | 0 g |
|---|---|
| 2 cups tossed lettuce and tomato salad | 5 g |
| **Asparagus or Green Beans Parmesan** | 5 g |
| **Total carbohydrates for Day 4** | **34.5 g** |

# DAY 5

### Breakfast

| Mushroom omelet made with 3 egg whites and 1 or 2 egg yolks and ½ cup sautéed onions and bell peppers | 5.5 g |
|---|---|
| 2 slices Canadian bacon | 0 g |
| Coffee with 1% milk and sweetener | 1.5 g |

### A.M. Snack

| 15 olives | 5 g |
|---|---|

### Lunch

| 1 cup onion soup | 5 g |
|---|---|
| 4 ounces shrimp salad (boiled shrimp, celery, onion, and 2 tablespoons mayo) served on bed of greens and radicchio | 5 g |

### P.M. Snack

| Celery spread with 1 ounce cream cheese | 1 g |
|---|---|

### Dinner

| **Chicken Mediterranean** | 4 g |
|---|---|
| 2 cups lettuce and tomato salad with **Creamy Vinaigrette** | 5 g |

D-Zerta gelatin topped with 2 tablespoons
   Cool Whip ............................................................... 2 g

**Total carbohydrates for Day 5**             **34 g**

# DAY

## Breakfast

2 poached eggs on Canadian bacon served on a bed
   of steamed spinach (½ cup) with 2 tablespoons
   **Hollandaise Sauce**, if desired       3 g
Coffee with 1% milk and sweetener      1.5 g

## A.M. Snack

¼ cup pistachio nuts (47 nuts)        5 g

## Lunch

4 cups spinach salad with 2 slices bacon crumbled,
   1 hard-cooked egg, and ¼ cup walnuts with
   **Vinaigrette** or other no-carb dressing     6 g

## P.M. Snack

2 ounces reduced fat cheese        2 g

## Dinner

Broiled lobster (1–1.5lb)         1 g
2 cups endive salad with no-carb dressing    2 g
Spaghetti squash, steamed, served with butter
   and Parmesan cheese         5 g
D-Zerta gelatin with 2 tablespoons Cool Whip   2 g

**Total carbohydrates for Day 6**       **27.5 g**

# 7 DAY

## Breakfast

| | |
|---|---:|
| 2 poached eggs | 1 g |
| 2 slices Canadian bacon | 0 g |
| ½ tomato, sliced, grilled if desired | 3 g |
| Coffee with 1% milk and sweetener | 1.5 g |

## A.M. Snack

| | |
|---|---:|
| 1 cup onion soup | 5 g |
| ¼ cup blueberries | 5 g |

## Lunch

| | |
|---|---:|
| 4 ounces broiled chicken (skinless) | 0 g |
| 1 cup cucumber, onion, and watercress salad with **Vinaigrette** or other no-carb dressing | 2 g |

## P.M. Snack

| | |
|---|---:|
| Roast beef, sliced and rolled | 0 g |

## Dinner

| | |
|---|---:|
| Tuna steak, broiled, dressed with ¼ cup salsa | 2 g |
| ½ cup **Coleslaw** | 5 g |
| Broccoli florets, steamed, with ½ teaspoon butter and squeeze of lemon juice | 3 g |
| **Total carbohydrates for Day 7** | **27.5 g** |

# RECIPES FOR CARBOHYDRATE COUNTERS

For your convenience, the recipes are listed in alphabetical order.

## ASPARAGUS OR GREEN BEANS PARMESAN

1–2 pounds asparagus or 2 cups green beans, whole, stemmed
1–2 tablespoons butter
    Salt
    Ground black pepper
⅓   cup grated Parmesan cheese (see note)

Place a steamer basket in a large pot with 1 inch of water. Bring to a boil over high heat. Place the asparagus or green beans in the basket, reduce the heat to medium and steam until almost ready to eat, 8 to 10 minutes. Rinse with cold water to prevent further cooking. Place in a buttered casserole dish. Dot with butter and add salt and pepper to taste. Top with ¼ cup of the cheese. Bake at 450°F until the cheese is just beginning to turn brown. Remove from the oven, sprinkle with the remaining cheese, and serve.

MAKES 4 SERVINGS
PER SERVING: 5 G CARBOHYDRATES

Note: If you are using fresh Parmesan cheese, I find that cutting it into thin slices with a potato peeler works better than grating it.

## CHICKEN MEDITERRANEAN

4   tablespoons olive oil
4   chicken thighs (skin removed)
1   onion, sliced
1   can (15 ounces) whole tomatoes

1 cup white wine
1 clove garlic, crushed
  Salt
  Ground black pepper
  Black olives (optional)

Heat the oil in a large saucepan over medium-high heat. Add the chicken and cook until browned. Remove from the saucepan. Add the onion to the same pan and cook until transparent but not brown. Add the tomatoes, wine, and garlic. Add salt and pepper to taste. Add the olives, if using. Replace the chicken back into the saucepan. Cover, reduce heat to low, and cook for 20 minutes, or until the chicken is cooked through.

MAKES 4 SERVINGS
PER SERVING: 4 G CARBOHYDRATES

## COLD TOMATOES STUFFED WITH SEAFOOD

4 firm unpeeled tomatoes
  Salt

STUFFING
1 can (6 ounces) tuna, crab, or shrimp (about ½ cup)
1 onion, chopped
1–2 ribs celery, chopped
1 green bell pepper, chopped
  Salt
  Ground black pepper
3 tablespoons mayonnaise
  Lettuce
  Vinaigrette (page 148)

Cut a cavity in the stem end of each of the tomatoes, sprinkle with salt, and invert on a rack to drain as you prepare the stuffing.

*To make the stuffing:* In a bowl, mix together the tuna, crab, or shrimp with the onion, celery, and bell pepper. Add salt and black pepper to taste. Add the mayonnaise (the mixture should be wet but not gooey).

Fill the tomatoes with the seafood salad and serve on a bed of lettuce lightly dressed with Vinaigrette.

MAKES 4 SERVINGS
PER SERVING: 6 G CARBOHYDRATES

# COLESLAW

| | |
|---|---|
| 1 | small head cabbage, thinly sliced |
| ⅔ | cup thinly sliced celery |
| ¼ | cup thinly sliced scallions |
| ½ | cup finely diced green bell pepper |
| 1 | small apple, peeled, cored, and finely sliced |
| 1 | medium cucumber, peeled, seeded, and thinly sliced |
| ½ | cup mayonnaise |
| ⅓ | cup sour cream |
| ½ | tablespoon Dijon mustard |
| 2 | tablespoons wine vinegar or cider vinegar |
| 1 | teaspoon salt |
| ¼ | teaspoon caraway seeds |
| ¼ | teaspoon celery seeds |
| | Ground black pepper |

In a large bowl, combine the cabbage, celery, scallions, bell pepper, apple, and cucumber. In a small bowl, mix the mayonnaise, sour cream, mustard, vinegar, salt, caraway seeds, and celery seeds. Mix into the cabbage mixture and add black pepper to taste.

MAKES 10 (½ CUP) SERVINGS
PER SERVING: 6 G CARBOHYDRATES

## CREAMY VINAIGRETTE

1    egg
¼    cup vinegar (see note)
1    teaspoon Dijon mustard
1    teaspoon shallots, minced
¾    cup olive oil
     Salt
     Ground black pepper

In a blender, combine the egg, vinegar, mustard, and shallots. Blend until smooth. With the blender running at a low speed, drizzle in the oil. When the mixture is creamy and quite thick, add salt and pepper to taste.

MAKES 12 SERVINGS (1 CUP)
PER SERVING: 1 G CARBOHYDRATES

Note: For the best flavor, use a good-quality vinegar. The mixture will thicken in the refrigerator. Add 1 to 2 teaspoons warm water to achieve the consistency you like.

## HOLLANDAISE SAUCE

1    stick butter
3    egg yolks
½    teaspoon salt
1    tablespoon lemon juice
     Pinch of mustard powder

Melt the butter in a saucepan over low heat, making sure it doesn't burn. In a blender, combine the egg yolks, salt, lemon juice, and mustard powder. With the blender running, drizzle in the melted butter. The mixture will thicken. Add more lemon juice or seasoning if desired. Use immediately or keep warm by putting it in a bowl and nesting the bowl in another bowl filled with very hot water. It will keep for up to 30 minutes this way.

MAKES 6 SERVINGS
PER SERVING: 0 G CARBOHYDRATES

# VINAIGRETTE

⅓  cup olive oil

⅓  cup wine vinegar (see note)

⅓  cup water

1–2 cloves garlic, minced

Salt

Ground black pepper

In a small bowl, mix the oil, vinegar, water, and garlic. Add salt and pepper to taste.

MAKES 6 SERVINGS
PER SERVING: 1 G CARBOHYDRATES

Note: You can replace up to half of the vinegar with mustard; Dijon mustard works best.

# CHAPTER 7

# THE COUNTING CALORIES DIET

CHANCES ARE YOU DON'T know my patient Janet, but then again, you've probably known someone like her. Or maybe you are that someone. Janet is 32. She works in a high-powered law firm in Washington, D.C., as a paralegal. She's divorced, with two children. Janet was pretty active as a kid and teenager. She loved sports, especially swimming and tennis. She was never skinny; she had broad shoulders and some real muscle. Although she was big, she never thought of herself as fat. After college came working 9 to 5, then marriage and two children. Suddenly, by her midtwenties, Janet found herself overweight. She wanted to lose weight, but she didn't really know how. She tried diets—lots of diets.

Janet's best success had come with a low-carbohydrate, high-protein diet. As a teenager she had lost weight with the Scarsdale diet. Then she'd tried the Atkins diet, the Protein Power diet, the Carbohydrate Addict's diet. They all worked for a while, but eventually she found herself gorging on bread and potatoes. She told me that at one point she felt as if she would kill for corn on the cob. She never felt hungry, it's true. But she never felt satisfied either. And without satisfaction, she couldn't stick to the diet, and she would revert to her old ways of eating.

The last few years she'd been trying the low-fat diets. They sounded healthier and allowed her the carbs she so loved. "I've Pritikined, I've Ornished, I've tried to Stop the Madness, but I couldn't. It just didn't work." On these diets, mealtime seemed to mean huge and depressing piles of salad or vegetables. And although she did get to eat the pasta and bread she wanted, she'd felt hungry, tired, and really, really cranky.

She came to me, she said, because she couldn't afford another "success" like she'd had in the past. "Another diet that ends up putting 20 pounds on me, and I just don't know what I'd do."

The traditional view of weight loss is that it's really just a little math problem: "Oh, if I eat 500 fewer calories, I'll lose a pound a week. Great." You wouldn't be reading this book if it were that easy.

It is true that reducing the number of calories you consume is an essential component of losing weight, and what *all* diets do is arrange what you eat so that you do, in fact, take in fewer calories. The trick to any successful diet is to eat fewer calories but to do it in a way that fools your body and brain into feeling that you are satisfied and never hungry. Low-fat diets try to do this by giving you unlimited amounts of fruits and vegetables and helping you fill up on real stick-to-the-ribs foods like pasta, grains, and starchy beans. Low-carb diets try to bore you to thinness by giving you access to all the meat you can eat, and betting that the satisfying aspect of meats and proteins and the monotony of the diet will help you to simply eat less of these high-calorie foods.

A diet that counts calories gets rid of these somewhat arbitrary limits on foods and allows you to eat all types of food. The trick in this diet—since they all have one—is to direct you to the foods that are the most satisfying and most filling from *all* food categories. By doing this, we can use the foods that work well in the low-fat diets and the low-carb diets, and we can satisfy one of the most basic needs we all have—the real need for variety in the foods we eat. A diet that explicitly tries to reduce calories can help many people lose weight. If you have filled out the questionnaire and arrived at this chapter, it is because you are one of those people.

In this chapter, we will look at who does well on a calorie-counting diet and which diet characteristics can make this way of eating successful. I have also provided a list of low-calorie foods and a 7-day eating plan. Finally, I've given you some simple recipes that can help you incorporate many of these principles into meals you can enjoy for a lifetime.

Who are the people who do well on, and what makes them compatible with, a low-calorie diet? First and foremost, these are individuals who need variety in their diets. Not everyone does. Some people eat the same thing for dinner 3 or 4 days a week and enjoy that. Breakfast, lunch, and dinner have a sameness, a familiarity that they enjoy. You are not one of those people. You crave variety in taste, in texture, in aroma, in richness. You've fallen off the diet wagon because of boredom and impatience with the unending sameness of the foods available to you.

In fact, monotony is one of the weight-loss tools used in many diets, though they probably won't tell you that. The same-old-same-old dampens appetite, at least for a time. Eventually, though, most of us crave the chance to eat something different at least every now and then. It is hardwired into us as a mechanism to ensure we get the full range of nutrients we need. For those folks who do well on a diet that looks only at calories, the variety and sensory qualities of foods are vital components of their satisfaction.

Do you find yourself at the end of the day standing in front of the refrigerator with the door open, looking for something crunchy or sour or aromatic or rich after the bland nourishments of a low-fat diet with all its veggies and pasta? Or do you crave the refreshing crispness of a partially ripe pear after a few days of steak and more steak on a low-carbohydrate diet? Then welcome to the Counting Calories Diet. This is where you belong.

*The Perfect Fit for David (lost 36 pounds)*
*I feel like I've been fighting my weight all my life. I was about to turn 55 and I thought, it's now or never. Oh, I've been on diets before. Lots of them. You name it. And I could lose the weight but I'd get bored (with the food), frustrated (with the restrictions), tired (of the work), and go back to the bad old ways. I had high blood pressure, high cholesterol, and metabolic syndrome. A couple of years ago I almost had a heart attack but I got a stent instead. Even after that, I couldn't lose the weight. This spring I had to have another stress test; it was fine but on that treadmill I decided—this is it. I have to win this potentially deadly battle of the bulge.*

*Keeping the diet diary was surprisingly easy for me. I like the routines in my life, so it was simple to add one more thing. I noticed a couple of things when I filled out the questionnaire. First, variety was essential to me. I was a Carnimore, sure, but I was also a VegeCarian, and a Starch Stealer and a Sweets Eater. I maxed out in every category. I needed variety. Of course, I guess I knew that about myself; I certainly never considered these monotonous diets that my friends had been on that try to bore you into losing weight. But I also needed volume, too. When I added it all up, I tied in the calorie-counting and fat-counting diets. I also saw that I had a tendency to binge eat—not too often, but enough to really throw my way of eating out of whack. I guess I knew that, but seeing it on paper really made it real.*

*The good news was that I exercised every day. In my own mind that was what was keeping me from having another heart attack.*

*Together with Dr. Sanders I came up with a plan that I thought would get the job done. It was the Counting Calories Diet, but with big servings of fruits and vegetables. Because I have metabolic syndrome, I got rid of most of the pastas and cut down on the bread and crackers. I gave myself nuts and low-fat cheeses for snacks; that kept me from getting hungry between meals and was a little treat. I had fruit with just about every meal to take the edge off my cravings for sweets and that worked remarkably well. In 6 months I went from 235 to 205. And it was practically painless. I'm never hungry, yet I only eat the foods I love.*

*Weekends were the toughest because my life was much less structured on those days. After church at the congregation's coffee hour, I had the greatest temptation because I'd be hungry and there was all this food around. All of it good, and very little of it was the kind of thing I'd want to eat: too much pastry, chips, little sandwiches. I figured out that if I had a snack right before church, I could pick through the offerings afterward in a sensible manner. Most weeks I don't eat any of it. If I'm going to choose my calories, I'm not going to waste them on foods I don't much care for.*

*My biggest challenge was a recent vacation in Ireland. Two weeks in a nation with plentiful ale and few vegetables. Stepping on the scale on my return confirmed what my clothes had already told me: I hadn't gained a pound. Now I'm under 200 and it feels good. My blood pressure is better; my cholesterol is the best it's been in years. I don't measure my portions, but I know they are smaller. The way I eat now fulfilled a lifelong goal; I get the pleasure I need from eating with a diet that is both healthy and sustainable. What more can I ask for?*

David, like Janet, is a classic calorie-counting dieter.

Why? First of all, they both craved variety in their diets. David already knew that about himself; Janet had to find out the hard way—through trial and failure. It was clear from their diet diaries and their diet histories that they craved variety in taste, texture, aroma, and richness. Janet had fallen off the diet wagon because of boredom with the unending sameness of the foods available to her. David wouldn't even try those types of diets. Variety was the key to their satisfaction, and only a low-calorie diet will allow them to choose from the full palette of foods.

Another important quality in these dieters was the recognition that more food was not what they wanted; what they craved was more kinds of foods. That is the essential trade-off in a low-calorie diet and is at the heart of its success. In a low-fat diet, you trade eating a high-calorie, high-fat food for the pleasure of eating more of a low-fat, low-calorie food. In a low-carb diet, you trade the volume of a high-carbohydrate diet for one rich in fats and proteins. In the low-calorie diet, you trade eating a lot of any single food for a chance to eat a little of a lot of different foods. This was a bargain David and Janet were willing to make. David wanted volume, but was able to satisfy that need with larger portions of the low-calorie fruits and vegetables that were at the heart of his diet. In exchange, he was willing to limit the portions of the other higher-calorie foods he enjoyed. He recognized that controlling portions had been essential and successful in his previous diets. Janet came to this from the other direction. She'd tried the all-you-can-eat-of-one-food diets and had come away wanting different food—not more food.

## THE BASICS OF A CALORIE-COUNTING DIET

You don't hear many people raving about their wildly successful calorie-counting diets these days. That's (in part) because if you cut calories willy-nilly, if you cut high-calorie foods and try to live only on low-calorie foods without choosing the foods that will help keep you feeling full, you will be hungry and will fail. This is the diet of iceberg lettuce with low-fat ranch dressing. This is the diet of tuna and Melba toast. They lack variety; they lack substance; they leave you hungry; they doom you to failure. A basic principle in dieting is that you must eat foods that you like and eat in a way that satisfies you, or you won't be able to stay on the diet. It's a law of nature almost as immutable as gravity. A smart low-calorie diet—one with smaller portions but greater pleasure—is the only way to make this principle work.

Recently, a couple of cereal companies recommended a low-calorie diet that featured their cereals prominently (naturally). The idea was to eat this diet cereal for breakfast and for lunch and then eat a normal dinner. Liquid diet products also advocated this type of calorie-restricted diet. Drink a can of diet meal replacement for breakfast and lunch and then eat a modest-size dinner at night. Here's the problem: There is no way that by the end of the day you are going to be able to eat a modest-size dinner. By the time you sit down to dinner, you are starving! And, if you are someone who craves variety, you haven't gotten any by the time you reach dinner.

These diets sell themselves as reasonable alternatives, but in fact they are virtually impossible to follow. And when you fail on them, do you blame the company for suggesting an unreasonable way to lose weight? No, chances are you fault yourself for a lack of willpower. I'm here to tell you that no one can stand up to real hunger. It goes against the way our bodies are put together. To succeed, you must choose foods that maximize your sense of fullness and satisfy the parts of you that need to be satisfied.

How can you do that?

First, on a low-calorie diet—or on any diet for that matter—you need to focus on foods that make you feel full and keep you feeling full until it's time for you to eat again. Each of the three food components—carbs, fats, and proteins—has an important role in making you feel full. Carbohydrates provide bulk or volume, especially those that are high in fiber and low in glycemic load. (If you aren't familiar with the concept of glycemic load, see page 124 for a crash course.) Your stomach is full—literally—and that helps you feel satisfied. High-fiber carbs also stay in your stomach longer, which makes that satisfaction last longer.

Proteins work somewhat differently. These foods are broken down into their component amino acids by digestive enzymes. These enzymes are released into your intestines only when proteins are eaten and disappear rapidly once the protein has been digested. In addition to their role in helping you make use of nutrients in proteins, several of these enzymes serve another, very important job: They communicate with your brain to let you know that you have eaten and that it was good. One of the many weight-loss drugs being tested by pharmaceutical companies is based on one of the most powerful of these enzymes known as CCK (cholecystokinin). And yet you can make this with stuff you have at home (in your stomach) for free, just by eating protein.

Fats are digested slowly. When you eat foods that contain a lot of fat, you are likely to feel full for longer simply because they hang around longer.

Because different foods work differently to make you feel full, each meal should be made up of proteins, complex carbohydrates, and some fat to maximize your sense of fullness. The real bonus of a calorie-counting diet is that you can eat all three types of foods based on what works best for you. The ideal proportion of these depends on the individual. You need to figure out what makes you full, but on a low-calorie diet I recommend eating a big portion of low-glycemic-load, high-fiber, unrefined carbohydrates (between 45 and 50 percent of the calories in a meal), and splitting the remainder between proteins (15 to 25 percent) and fats (35 to 40 percent). David ended up with a diet that is high in non-starchy carbohydrates and low-saturated-fat meats, nuts, and cheeses. Janet realized that pasta was essential to her satiety, but that she was able to manage her weight if she made her pasta dishes with equal parts pasta and veggies and a little meat—just for the flavor.

Here's another important point to remember while following a calorie-counting diet: You must eat when you are hungry, not when you are starving. If you allow yourself to get really, really hungry, it becomes very difficult to make yourself stop once you finally get a chance to eat. This is true no matter what diet you are following, but it takes on particular importance in a calorie-counting diet, because portion control is such an important aspect of the diet.

Moreover, when you are really hungry, it is virtually impossible to resist any temptation. If you pass on a bowl of chocolates or chips when you are starving, the chance that you will be able to just walk on by drops dramatically. Your ability to pass the McDonald's or the bakery on your way home is also impaired. You might be able to do it much of the time—though it's hard work—but you won't be able to do it *all* of the time. So plan to have three meals a day as well as one or two snacks. This way, you will increase your chances of eating what you should eat and responding to the body's cues when you have eaten enough.

A third strategy for a successful calorie-counting diet: Try to eat most of your calories early in the day. Breakfast should contain around one-third of the calories you are planning to eat that day. This is a more natural way to eat—providing your body with the fuel it needs to take on the day—and it maximizes your body's ability to burn the calories you take in over the course of the day. It also sends you into the evening with less hunger, and that's important, because the social aspect of dinner makes it an ideal opportunity to overeat. It's a lot easier to pass up that opportunity if you are hungry but not starving when dinnertime comes around.

Try to eat a variety of foods, tastes, and textures at every meal since, if you are reading this chapter, chances are that variety is an important signal of satisfaction. Maximize the satiety signals you send your body by providing yourself with the variety you crave.

## PORTION: THE KEY TO SUCCESS

The final aspect of a low-calorie diet that needs to be discussed is portion size. Thanks to the supersize world we live in, our sense of portion size is way out of control. When you start eating huge portions that have too many calories, you're likely to feel uncomfortable at first, even sick. But after a surprisingly short time, you get used to that portion size, and if you get less, you feel that the smaller portion is too small. Your eyes get used to seeing a certain amount of food on the plate as a visual cue to how much is enough. Your eyes accommodate to different portion sizes quickly—much more quickly than your stomach—and you learn to eat bigger (or, more rarely, smaller) portions quite easily.

But this is the world we find ourselves in: We crave variety, and voilà!—it's there, 24/7. We crave big steaming portions that fill up bigger and bigger plates. We get that, too. And we have foods that are targeted to our most primeval needs: lots of fat, lots of carbs—throw in some salt, and you're in heaven. That is a diet for widespread obesity. America is on such a diet. And it's working.

Our job is to figure out a way to eat in this world so that our bodies look and act the way we want them to, not the way fast-food corporations want them to. That's what this book is all about. We live in a culture where we can eat pretty much anything we want, whenever we want, and as much as we want. It's up to us to decide how to eat.

So, does a low-calorie diet work? Just ask David. He lost over 35 pounds since he started eating this way, and he's still going strong. And Janet has neared her target size. She's actually had to buy a whole new wardrobe. It worked for them; it could work for you, too.

## THE PERFECT FIT COUNTING CALORIES BASIC DIET

In a diet that focuses on counting calories, there are really only two questions: how many and what? Specifically, how many calories you should eat per day and what foods will make up those calories. Let's start with how many. I recommend that most people start with a 1,200-calorie diet. Before you roll your eyes and grab your stomach, let me tell you why. Our bodies are designed to love staying the same. We hate change at the most basic level. You can see this with weight gain, even though we are purposefully designed to gain weight more easily than we lose weight. Most people have to overeat for several days (and for some lucky few, even weeks) before they see a change in the way their clothes fit or notice a change on the scale. Our bodies seek stability; if the body can avoid change, it does. Research has shown us over and over again that you can increase the number of calories in a person's diet, and he or she will maintain the same weight—although not for too long.

It's the same thing with weight loss. If you reduce your calories by 500 calories a day (basically, one bagel or two colas less per day), then theoretically you would lose a pound in 7 days. That's the theory; the reality is that because our bodies resist change, you don't lose that pound. Physics says you will; but our bodies give a raspberry to physics, at least for a while. We resist weight gain by increasing (ever so slightly) our metabolism. We resist weight loss by decreasing (again, ever so slightly) our metabolism. Moreover, if you eliminate those calories while maintaining the same essential diet—except for the foods you are cutting out—you will probably get hungry, and you may not be able to consistently get rid of those 500 calories. So if you cut back your diet by 500 calories, you will lose weight, but it may take a while for that change to make itself known on the scale or in your clothes.

To get around this little obstacle, I put most of my patients on a 1,200-calorie diet to get things started. At 1,200 calories, you probably will see a 1- to 2-pound weight change per week, and chances are, if you follow the diet and eat foods that will fill your stomach and satisfy your need for variety, you will be able to eat those paltry (you think) 1,200 calories and not get hungry.

Who shouldn't be on a 1,200-calorie-a-day diet? If you really stick to the diet and find that you are hungry, then you should consider increasing your daily calorie intake to 1,500 calories a day. Most of my patients do well on a 1,200-calorie-a-day diet. A few, mostly men, have needed 1,500 calories a day; a couple who were very overweight have needed 1,800 calories. But, in general, most can tolerate this level of calorie reduction pretty well.

I recommend that you try the 1,200 calories for 4 to 5 days. Make sure you are eating three meals a day; make sure you are snacking; make sure you are eating foods from each of the three food types (proteins, carbohydrates, and fats). And if you find that you are still unsatisfied, up the calorie content by 300 calories. If you still feel hungry, up it again. You won't be able to follow a diet if you are hungry, so increase the calorie content until you are comfortable and feel satisfied but not overly full at the end of each meal. Another tip, if you are not hungry for your next snack or meal, then you probably ate too much at your last meal. When that happens, reduce your portion even more.

Now, what should you be eating? Lots of carbohydrates, certainly. These should be high-fiber, low-glycemic-load carbs. What that really means is that you will be eating plenty of fruits and vegetables, some whole-grain bread, and some pastas and rice. You will see from the 7-day eating plan that almost half of your calories will come from foods like this. You will be eating lots of dairy products—the low-fat variety, since the fat in most dairy products is saturated and promotes heart disease in many people. You will be eating meat, poultry, or fish every day. Again, I encourage you to choose the low-fat versions of these foods, because the fats contained in them are primarily saturated fats. You won't be avoiding fat—up to 40 percent of your calories will come from fat—but it will be primarily mono- and polyunsaturated fat (from olive oil and nuts) and omega fats (from fish).

To make this work, it's important to keep a food diary. Write down everything you eat and drink. I think I've convinced you that it's hard to know what you eat unless you write it down. Now that you are changing the way you eat, it's more important than ever. I also recommend that you measure everything you eat, at least initially. You might think you know how much you are eating, but I bet if you measured it out you would be surprised. You will learn pretty quickly what half a cup looks like and how much meat makes up a 4-ounce serving, so you won't have to do this forever. But you should weigh and measure everything for the first week of this eating plan.

You will notice that I have not included very many preprocessed foods. That's because most of those foods include fats, salt, and sugar as preservatives. These are empty calories. Some folks call candy empty calories because it provides sweets without any other nutrients. I think there is a place for sweets in a balanced diet. But calories that are added just to make the food last longer on the shelf or in the freezer are the truly empty calories. They work for the manufacturer, but not for you. Moreover, many processed foods—particularly baked goods like breads, pastries, and muffins—contain trans fats. Trans fats promote heart disease and are found in only tiny amounts in unprocessed foods. Manufacturers developed these fats to replace butter but did too good a job. It turns out that they act very much like butter in your system, so just leave them out of your diet. (If you want to know more about saturated fat, like butter, and trans fats, see chapter 9.)

On this low-calorie diet, you should lose 1 to 2 pounds per week. If after 2 weeks you haven't lost weight, check your diary to see what you have been eating. Have you eaten unplanned foods? Which ones? Why did you eat them? Is there any way to fit them in without blowing your calorie cap? And what about your portion sizes—are you measuring? Have they crept up? Finally, consider the possibility that 1,200 calories are too many for you. I have several patients who needed to reduce their intake to 1,000 calories per day. This is a science experiment, and you are the test tube. No one can tell you exactly what to eat to make yourself feel good and weigh the right amount. In the final analysis, you have to figure out what makes you feel good and how to eat that way. I'm simply here to help.

Below I've listed some foods that could be part of a low-calorie diet, and I've listed them in amounts that will give you 100 calories. That could be 1½ medium-size artichokes or 5 crackers. I've listed them in categories: protein, carbs, and fats. You need to eat some from each column in order to maximize your feeling of fullness. Nearly half of your calories will probably come from carbohydrates (fruits, vegetables, starches), up to 20 percent of your calories will come from proteins (meats, poultry, seafood, dairy products, and nuts), and 35 to 40 percent of your calories will come from fats. I've also provided a 7-day eating plan to let you see how you might put all this together. I end this chapter with a few recipes that have been helpful to my patients and to me. In fact, David and Janet both have given me recipes that they have found helpful in their new way of eating.

## SIX TIPS FOR CALORIE COUNTERS

1. Eat foods that make you feel full: carbs that contain fiber and have a low glycemic load; low-fat (lower-calorie) proteins; and some amount of fat. You must eat all three in each meal or snack.

2. Eat when you are hungry, not when you are starving.

3. Get your calories in early—breakfast is a must; try to have at least two-thirds of your calories before dinner.

4. Variety can mean more work, but it's a powerful satisfier. Don't skimp on sources of satisfaction.

5. Portion size is key; measure your portions until you know what you are eating.

6. Keep a diet diary—knowledge is power.

# FOOD LIST FOR THE COUNTING CALORIES BASIC DIET

| Proteins | 100-Calorie Portion |
|---|---|

**MEAT, POULTRY, AND SEAFOOD** (4 ounces is considered a normal serving size, and this assumes that meats are cooked without adding fats.)

**BEEF**

| | |
|---|---|
| Chuck roast (pot roast) | 1½ oz |
| London broil | 2 oz |
| Sirloin steak, lean only | 1.7 oz |

**PORK**

| | |
|---|---|
| Bacon | 2 slices |
| Canadian bacon | 2½ oz |
| Ham | 1½ oz |
| Pork chop | 2 oz |

**POULTRY**

| | |
|---|---|
| Chicken, no skin | 2 oz |
| Chicken, with skin | 1½ oz |
| Turkey, no skin | 3 oz |
| Turkey, with skin | 2 oz |

**SEAFOOD**

| | |
|---|---|
| Clams | 4 oz/8 clams |
| Flounder | 3 oz |
| Oysters | 3 oz/10 oysters |
| Salmon, fresh | 2 oz |
| Salmon, smoked | 3 oz |
| Shrimp (medium) | 4 oz/16 shrimp |
| Tuna, fresh | 2½ oz |
| Tuna, water-packed | 2 oz |

## CHEESE

| | |
|---|---|
| American | 1 oz/1 slice |
| American, low-fat | 2 oz/2 slices |
| Cheddar, low-fat | 2 oz |
| Colby, low-fat | 2 oz |
| Feta | 1½ oz |
| Mozzarella | 1 oz |
| Mozzarella, low-fat | 1½ oz |
| Parmesan | 1 oz |
| String cheese | 1 oz |
| Swiss | 1 oz |

## DAIRY

| | |
|---|---|
| Eggs | 1 jumbo/2 small |
| Milk, fat-free | 1½ cups |
| Milk, 1% | 1 cup |
| Milk, whole | ⅔ cup |

## NUTS

| | |
|---|---|
| Almonds | ½ oz/15 whole kernels |
| Cashews | ½ oz |
| Peanuts, roasted | ½ oz |
| Pecans | ½ oz/10 halves |
| Pistachio nuts | ½ oz/20 nuts |

| Carbohydrates | 100-Calorie Portion |
|---|---|

## VEGETABLES

| | |
|---|---|
| Artichoke, fresh | 1½ medium globes |
| Asparagus, canned | 2 cups/33 spears |
| Asparagus, fresh | 25 spears |
| Avocado, fresh | ⅓ medium |
| Beans, green, fresh | 2 cups/approx. 50 whole |

| | |
|---|---|
| Beans, kidney, canned | ½ cup |
| Beans, lima | ½ cup |
| Beets | 1½ cups |
| Black-eyed peas | 1 cup |
| Broccoli | 2 cups |
| Brussels sprouts | 1½ cups |
| Cabbage | ½ head |
| Carrots, fresh | 5 large whole |
| Cauliflower | ½ head/30 florets |
| Celery | 10 whole ribs/5 cups strips |
| Corn | ½ cup |
| Cucumber | 2½ whole |
| Eggplant, peeled | 1 medium |
| Lentils | ½ cup |
| Lettuce | 1 large head |
| Peas, field | ½ cup |
| Peas, green | 2 cups |
| Peas, snow or sugar snap | 1½ cups |
| Peppers, bell | 4 whole |
| Potato, baked | ½ medium |
| Potato, sweet | 1 medium |
| Spinach | 10 cups |
| Squash, acorn | 1 cup |
| Squash, yellow or zucchini | 3 cups |
| Tomato, canned | 1 cup |
| Tomato, fresh | 5 medium |
| Yam | ¾ cup |

## FRUITS

| | |
|---|---|
| Apple | 1 cup/1 large |
| Apricot | 1⅓ cups/5 whole |
| Banana | 1 medium |
| Blueberries | ½ cup/120 berries |

| | |
|---|---|
| Figs | 2 whole |
| Grapefruit | 1 cup/1 whole |
| Grapes | 1 cup/25 pieces |
| Kiwifruit | 2 whole |
| Mango | 1 cup/1 small |
| Melon, cantaloupe | ½ medium |
| Nectarines | 1 whole |
| Peaches | 2 medium |
| Pears | 1 medium |
| Plums | 3 whole |
| Raisins | 75 pieces |
| Raspberries | ½ pint/1½ cups |
| Strawberries | 20 medium berries |
| Tangerines | 2 whole |
| Watermelon | ¾-inch slice large melon |

## BREADS AND PASTA

| | |
|---|---|
| Bagel, plain | ⅓ bagel |
| English muffin | ⅔ muffin |
| Garlic bread | 1 slice |
| Muffin, corn or bran | ½ muffin |
| Oatmeal bread | 1½ slices |
| Pasta (recommended serving size is 2 oz) | 1 oz |
| Raisin bread | 1 slice |
| Wheat bread | 1½ slices |
| Wheat bread, low-calorie | 2½ slices |
| White bread | 1½ slices |
| White bread, thin | 2 slices |
| Whole-grain bread | 1½ slices |

## CEREALS

| | |
|---|---|
| All-Bran | ¾ cup |
| All-Bran Extra Fiber | 1 cup |

| | |
|---|---|
| Cracklin' Oat Bran | ⅓ cup |
| Fiber One | 1 cup |
| 40% Bran Flakes | ⅔ cup |
| Frosted Mini Wheats | ⅔ cup |
| Granola | ¼ cup |
| Oatmeal, plain | ¾ cup |
| 100% bran | ½ cup |
| Raisin bran | ½ cup |
| Wheat Chex | 1 cup |

## CRACKERS

| | |
|---|---|
| Cheez-It | 20 crackers |
| Finn Crisp | 5 crackers |
| Goldfish | 1 oz |
| Melba toast | 6 crackers |
| Ritz | 6 crackers |
| RyKrisp | 3 crackers |
| Saltines | 8 crackers |
| Wheat Thins | 9 crackers |

## SPICES AND CONDIMENTS

| | |
|---|---|
| Ketchup | ¼ cup |
| Salsa | ¾ cup |
| Sugar | 8 tsp |
| Syrup | 2 tbsp |

| Fats | 100-Calorie Portion |
|---|---|

## OILS AND SPREADS

| | |
|---|---|
| Butter | 1 tbsp |
| Corn oil | 2 tsp |
| Mayonnaise | 1 tbsp |
| Olive oil | 2 tsp |
| Peanut butter | 1 tbsp |

## 1,200-CALORIE DAILY MEAL PLANS FOR THE COUNTING CALORIES DIET

(Dishes in **bold print** are listed alphabetically in the recipe section at the end of the chapter on page 176.)

# DAY 1

### Breakfast

| | |
|---|---|
| ¾ cup Fiber One (or some other high-fiber cereal) | 90 |
| ½ cup fat-free milk | 45 |
| ¼ cantaloupe | 50 |
| 1 slice low-calorie wheat bread | 40 |
| 1 tablespoon peanut butter | 95 |
| Total calories | 320 |

### A.M. Snack

| | |
|---|---|
| 1 plum | 40 |
| 1 Mozzarella cheese stick | 80 |
| Total calories | 120 |

### Lunch

| | |
|---|---|
| 1 cup chicken and rice soup | 75 |
| 2 cups mixed lettuce salad with tomatoes and cucumbers dressed with 1 tablespoon **Roquefort Sour Cream Dressing** | 200 |
| 2 Finn Crisp crackers | 40 |
| Total calories | 315 |

### P.M. Snack

| | |
|---|---|
| 2 cups microwave butter-flavored popcorn | 75 |
| Total calories | 75 |

## Dinner

| | |
|---|---|
| 1 boneless chicken cutlet (4 ounces), dredged in mixture of Parmesan cheese and bread crumbs, sautéed briefly in olive oil | 300 |
| 1 cup asparagus | 30 |
| 1 tomato, sliced | 15 |
| 1 cup raspberries with 2 tablespoons Cool Whip | 85 |
| Total calories | 430 |
| **Total calories for Day 1** | **1,260** |

# DAY

## Breakfast

| | |
|---|---|
| ⅔ cup oatmeal (not instant) with sweetener (not sugar) and ¼ cup 1% milk | 125 |
| 2 slices Canadian bacon | 90 |
| ½ cup blueberries | 40 |
| Total calories | 255 |

## A.M. Snack

| | |
|---|---|
| 8 ounces fat-free yogurt | 100 |
| Total calories | 100 |

## Lunch

| | |
|---|---|
| ½ cup black bean soup | 55 |
| 2 slices ham on low-calorie bread with lettuce, tomato, and 1 teaspoon each mayo and mustard | 230 |
| Total calories | 285 |

## P.M. Snack

| | |
|---|---:|
| 1 cup cut carrots and celery | 50 |
| 3 tablespoons hummus | 105 |
| Total calories | 155 |

## Dinner

| | |
|---|---:|
| 1 small steamed lobster dipped in butter (can substitute more veggies for butter and forget the dipping) | 250 |
| 1 medium artichoke | 60 |
| ½ tomato and ½ cucumber, sliced, with 1 tablespoon **Vinaigrette** | 75 |
| 1 light ice cream sandwich (Skinny Cow or Weight Watchers) | 100 |
| Total calories | 485 |
| **Total calories for Day 2** | **1,280** |

# DAY

## Breakfast

| | |
|---|---:|
| Breakfast sandwich (½ English muffin, 1 poached egg, 1 slice Canadian bacon, 1 slice American cheese) | 235 |
| ¼ cantaloupe | 50 |
| Total calories | 285 |

## A.M. Snack

| | |
|---|---:|
| ½ cucumber, sliced, with ½ cup low-fat cottage cheese | 100 |
| Total calories | 100 |

## Lunch

| | |
|---|---|
| 1 cup cream of asparagus soup (made with water) | 85 |
| 1 tomato stuffed with **Tuna and Corn Salad** | 225 |
| Total calories | 310 |

## P.M. Snack

| | |
|---|---|
| 2 plums | 70 |
| Total calories | 70 |

## Dinner

| | |
|---|---|
| **Chicken Mediterranean** | 385 |
| 1 cup green beans | 40 |
| 1 FrozFruit bar | 60 |
| Total calories | 485 |
| **Total calories for Day 3** | **1,250** |

# DAY

## Breakfast

| | |
|---|---|
| 1 slice watermelon | 100 |
| 1 slice cheese toast with tomato (1 slice low-calorie bread, 2 slices tomato, 1 slice American, Swiss, or low-fat Cheddar cheese with a smear of mustard) | 130 |
| Total calories | 230 |

## A.M. Snack

| | |
|---|---|
| Small **Fruit Smoothie** (½ serving) | 155 |
| Total calories | 155 |

## Lunch

| | |
|---|---:|
| Open-faced sandwich of low-calorie bread, 4 ounces sliced turkey, tomato, and lettuce with ½ tablespoon mayonnaise | 270 |
| ½ cup grapes (approx. 12) | 30 |
| Total calories | 300 |

## P.M. Snack

| | |
|---|---:|
| 2 cups microwave butter-flavored popcorn | 75 |
| Total calories | 75 |

## Dinner

| | |
|---|---:|
| 3 ounces broiled tuna, seasoned with 3 tablespoons salsa | 225 |
| 1 cup spinach, sautéed with garlic in olive oil | 50 |
| ½ cup steamed baby carrots | 35 |
| ½ cup fruit sorbet | 200 |
| Total calories | 510 |
| **Total calories for Day 4** | **1,270** |

# DAY 5

## Breakfast

| | |
|---|---:|
| 1 cup raisin bran with ½ cup fat-free milk | 235 |
| 1 slice low-calorie bread with 1 tablespoon peanut butter | 135 |
| Total calories | 370 |

## A.M. Snack

| | |
|---|---:|
| 1 cup turkey vegetable soup | 72 |
| Total calories | 72 |

## Lunch

| | |
|---|---|
| **Greek Salad** | 160 |
| 2 RyKrisp crackers | 60 |
| ¼ cantaloupe | 50 |
| Total calories | 270 |

## P.M. Snack

| | |
|---|---|
| 1 tangerine | 40 |
| Total calories | 40 |

## Dinner

| | |
|---|---|
| 1 serving **Pork Chops with Sweet Potatoes and Apples** | 320 |
| 1 medium artichoke | 60 |
| 1 cup raspberries with 2 tablespoons Cool Whip | 100 |
| Total calories | 480 |
| **Total calories for Day 5** | **1,232** |

# DAY 6

## Breakfast

| | |
|---|---|
| Omelet made with 1 whole egg and 2 additional egg whites, and 1 cup chopped green pepper, onion, and tomato | 170 |
| ½ cup **Ambrosia** | 100 |
| Total calories | 270 |

## A.M. Snack

| | |
|---|---|
| 2 figs | 75 |
| 1 ounce prosciutto ham | 50 |
| Total calories | 125 |

### Lunch

| | |
|---|---|
| 1 cup Manhattan clam chowder | 80 |
| 1 small baked potato stuffed with salsa and 2 tablespoons fat-free sour cream | 250 |
| ¼ cantaloupe | 50 |
| Total calories | 380 |

### P.M. Snack

| | |
|---|---|
| 12 almonds | 85 |
| Total calories | 85 |

### Dinner

| | |
|---|---|
| 12 medium boiled shrimp | 75 |
| Cocktail sauce (¼ cup ketchup mixed with horseradish) | 30 |
| 1 ear corn on the cob (no butter) | 125 |
| 1 cup steamed broccoli | 50 |
| 1 cup sliced strawberries with 2 tablespoons Cool Whip | 75 |
| Total calories | 355 |
| **Total calories for Day 6** | **1,215** |

# DAY 7

### Breakfast

| | |
|---|---|
| **Fruit Smoothie** | 310 |
| 1 slice low-calorie bread, toasted | 40 |
| 1 tablespoon peanut butter | 95 |
| Total calories | 445 |

## A.M. Snack

| | |
|---|---|
| ¼ cantaloupe | 50 |
| Total calories | 50 |

## Lunch

| | |
|---|---|
| 1 head endive and 1 tomato, sliced, dressed with **Avocado Dressing** | 245 |
| 2 Finn Crisp crackers | 40 |
| 1 tangerine | 40 |
| Total calories | 325 |

## P.M. Snack

| | |
|---|---|
| 2 cups microwave butter-flavored popcorn | 75 |
| Total calories | 75 |

## Dinner

| | |
|---|---|
| 4 ounces fat-free ham, heated in microwave oven | 120 |
| **Winter Squash Supreme** | 200 |
| 15 spears asparagus | 50 |
| Total calories | 370 |
| **Total calories for Day 7** | **1,265** |

# RECIPES FOR CALORIE COUNTERS

For your convenience, the recipes are listed in alphabetical order.

## AMBROSIA

2   oranges, halved
1   banana, sliced
½   cup shredded unsweetened coconut

Peel and thinly slice 3 of the orange halves. In a bowl, combine the sliced oranges, banana, and coconut. Juice the remaining orange half and pour the juice over the fruit mixture. Let sit for 5 to 10 minutes before serving.

MAKES 2 SERVINGS
PER SERVING: 200 CALORIES

## AVOCADO DRESSING

¼   avocado, peeled and mashed
2   tablespoons vinegar
½   teaspoon Dijon mustard
¼   cup olive oil

In a small bowl, combine the avocado, vinegar, and mustard. Drizzle in the oil while stirring. Mix well. Use immediately.

MAKES 4 SERVINGS (½ CUP)
PER SERVING: 110 CALORIES

## CHICKEN MEDITERRANEAN

4   tablespoons olive oil
4   chicken thighs
1   onion, sliced
1   can (15 ounces) whole tomatoes
1   cup white wine
1   clove garlic, crushed
    Salt
    Ground black pepper
    Black olives (optional)

Heat the oil in a large saucepan over medium-high heat. Add the chicken and cook until browned. Remove from the saucepan. Add the onion to the same pan and cook until transparent but not brown. Add the tomatoes, wine, and garlic. Add salt and pepper to taste. Add the olives, if using. Replace the chicken in the saucepan. Cover, reduce the heat to low, and cook for 20 minutes, or until the chicken is cooked through.

MAKES 4 SERVINGS
PER SERVING: 385 CALORIES

## FRUIT SMOOTHIE

I add a little All-Bran to my smoothies—I love it; others don't. Try it and see.

1   cup 1% milk
¼   cup plain yogurt
1   large ripe banana or other soft fruit, such as canned
       peaches or fresh or frozen berries
2–3 ice cubes
1   tablespoon All-Bran cereal (optional)

In a blender, combine the milk, yogurt, banana or other fruit, ice cubes, and cereal, if desired. Blend until smooth.

MAKES 1 SERVING
PER SERVING: 310 CALORIES

# GREEK SALAD

SALAD

4   cups lettuce, washed and shredded, or half lettuce and half spinach

1   medium tomato, cut into wedges

½   small onion, thinly sliced

2   ounces low-fat feta cheese, crumbled

6   Greek olives, pitted

DRESSING

¼   cup red wine

1   tablespoon olive oil

1   tablespoon dried oregano

2   teaspoons lemon juice

1   teaspoon fresh basil, chopped, or ½ teaspoon dried basil

*To make the salad:* In a large bowl, combine the lettuce or lettuce-spinach mixture with the tomato, onion, cheese, and olives.

*To make the dressing:* In a small bowl, mix the wine, oil, oregano, lemon juice, and basil. Add to the salad and toss to mix.

MAKES 1 SERVING
PER SERVING: 160 CALORIES

## PORK CHOPS WITH SWEET POTATOES AND APPLES

3   tablespoons all-purpose flour
    Salt
    Ground black pepper
2   pork chops, 3 ounces each
¼   cup diced onion
½–1 cup chicken broth
¼   cup apple cider
1   small sweet potato, sliced
1   apple, sliced

In a shallow bowl, mix the flour with salt and pepper to taste and dredge the pork chops in the flour mixture.

Heat a large nonstick skillet sprayed with olive oil over medium-high heat. Add the pork chops and cook for about 2 minutes on each side or until brown. Remove from the skillet and set aside.

In the same skillet, combine the onion and a small amount of the chicken broth. Cook until the onion is tender and translucent. Add the cider and more chicken broth. Add the sweet potato and allow to simmer for 5–8 minutes. Then add apples and pork chops. Cover, reduce heat, and simmer 5–10 minutes until the sweet potato and apple are tender. Add broth as needed to keep mixture moist but not soupy.

MAKES 2 SERVINGS
PER SERVING: 320 CALORIES

## ROQUEFORT SOUR CREAM DRESSING

¼   pound Roquefort or blue cheese
1   cup low-fat sour cream
1   tablespoon vinegar
1   tablespoon finely chopped onion or chives

Salt

Ground black pepper

In a blender, combine the cheese, sour cream, vinegar, and onion or chives. Blend to the desired consistency. Add salt and pepper to taste.

Makes 6 servings
Per serving: 55 calories

## TUNA AND CORN SALAD

1    cup corn, fresh or frozen, cooked; or canned, drained
1    can (6 ounces) water-packed tuna
3    ribs celery, chopped
½    onion, finely chopped
½    cup low-fat mayonnaise
    Pimientos
    Salt
    Ground black pepper

This recipe tastes best with fresh corn. Cook it in a microwave oven for 2 to 3 minutes, then cut it off the cob. If using frozen corn, cook it in a microwave oven for 1 minute, then rinse with cold water.

In a bowl, mix together the corn, tuna, celery, onion, and mayonnaise. Add the pimientos and salt and pepper to taste.

Makes 4 servings
Per serving: 190 calories

## VINAIGRETTE

⅓    cup olive oil
⅓    cup wine vinegar (see note)
⅓    cup water
1–2 cloves garlic, minced

Salt

Ground black pepper

In a small bowl, mix the oil, vinegar, water, and garlic. Add salt and pepper to taste.

MAKES 12 SERVINGS (1 CUP)
PER SERVING: 35 CALORIES

Note: You can replace up to half of the vinegar with mustard; Dijon mustard works best.

## WINTER SQUASH SUPREME

2   tablespoons olive oil
1   small butternut squash, cut into bite-size chunks
1   apple, cut into bite-size chunks, peeled if you like
⅓   bag (12 ounces) fresh cranberries
2   tablespoons brown sugar

Heat the oil in a large skillet over medium-high heat. Add the squash and cook, stirring frequently, for 5 to 7 minutes, or until it starts to soften. Add the apple. Cook together for another 5 minutes, then add the cranberries and brown sugar. Cook until everything is tender and the cranberries are swollen and soft.

MAKES 2 SERVINGS
PER SERVING: 200 CALORIES

# 8 CHAPTER
# THE COUNTING FATS DIET

UNTIL VERY RECENTLY, IF you went to your doctor and said you wanted to lose weight, he would hand you some pamphlets about a low-fat, high-carbohydrate diet. That was the only eating option offered by doctors, nutritionists, and for many years, even women's magazines. And while many doctors continue to plug the old standby, few books and checkout-counter journals tout that weight-loss strategy today.

Your grandmother's diet could use a good public-relations agent. It's struggling as it competes with the South Beach diet, the Carbohydrate Addict's diet, and the Peanut Butter diet. While there are a dozen different versions of the Zone diet and the Atkins diet, low-fat diets, with their exhortations to "Eat More and Weigh Less" or to "Stop the Madness," have practically disappeared from magazine covers and faded to the background of bookstore shelves.

So, can you lose weight on a low-fat diet? Or was it, as one recent story in *The New York Times Magazine* proclaimed, "A Big Fat Lie"? It was no lie. But in the jumble of America's ongoing gabfest about dieting, it always seems that the new idea disproves the old one. It doesn't, of course, and that's the main point of this book. Each of these eating regimens works, but it depends on who the dieter is and how well the plan is customized to the individual eater. The fact is, there have been hundreds of studies done on low-fat diets documenting their effectiveness. By one analysis, every 2 percent drop in the amount of fat you eat is associated with a 1-pound weight loss.

Successful dieters also testify to the effectiveness of a low-fat diet. In a survey of 4,000 men and women who had lost at least 30 pounds and maintained that weight loss for more than 5 years, many swore by a low-fat diet as the strategy they used to lose weight, and for virtually all it was a key component to how they maintained their new weight.

The big problem with the low-fat diet was that, until recently, it was the only diet available. Everyone got put on this diet, regardless of how they ate, how they lived, and what made them satisfied. It was the original, the officially sanctioned one-size-fits-all diet.

When that happened the failure rate for the low-fat diet, of course, soared. Sure, lots of folks were able to lose weight, but many more were not. And because it was considered the "right" way to eat, the failures were even more likely to be seen as a moral failing rather than a simple mismatch between dieter and diet.

Moreover, all fat became the "enemy." Because of this new way of thinking, the difference between "good" fats and "bad" fats was lost, and the important role that fat plays in any diet was forgotten.

As a result, this very effective approach to weight loss has been virtually abandoned—not by doctors and nutritionists, but by dieters who chalk it up to just one more failed diet strategy.

So who is this diet right for? Like all diets, that will depend on your food preferences, the ways in which you get full, your medical history, and your lifestyle. To figure out whether you should use a low-fat diet, you'll need to understand the basics of how one works—in other words, which fats to keep, which to get rid of, and, perhaps most important, which foods you can use to keep you from missing fats once you cut them down to size. This is the key feature that often makes low-fat diets fail: You must fashion a diet that will help you lose weight and yet allow you to feel satisfied. If you are suffering as you diet, then that diet won't work. Once you understand how a proper low-fat diet works, we'll move to a list of foods containing 5 grams of fat or less and a 7-day eating plan so you can see how to put these principles into action. Finally, at the end of the chapter, I have provided recipes that will give you some fresh ideas on how to cook and eat when you are counting fats.

Let's start with a look at the successful low-fat dieter.

## DIANE'S STORY

Diane is an attractive, 44-year-old woman who came to me when it looked to her as if it were inevitable that she would end up as big and round as her mother and her two older sisters. She is almost 6 feet tall, and so the weight she carried, just over 200 pounds, made her look tall and shapely, not at all fat. But over the past several years, her weight kept creeping upward. Her son, Matthew, now 7, had left her 15 pounds heavier than what she thought was her best weight, 160, and since her separation 2 years before, the scale seemed to move in only one direction. She was frustrated and a little angry.

"It's just not fair," she told me. "Okay, I'm not perfect. But mostly I eat right. Sometimes, though, I do eat too much, and when that happens, I feel like I put on the pounds and then they just never come off. It's not fair!"

We talked about her life and her diet. During the week, it was very hectic at her house; frequently, she was too busy to eat breakfast. Those days she might grab a donut and coffee after dropping off the kids on the way to work. For lunch, she and the other women at her office went to a neighborhood deli and got sandwiches—and the tasty homemade chips that went with them.

Dinner was erratic. The older child liked only sandwiches, and the younger one ate only macaroni and cheese. Once the kids were in bed, she often ate dinner standing at the refrigerator, picking at the leftovers from the weekend or from the pasta she made for her daughter. Diane's scheduled meals were small, but what she didn't eat at mealtime she ate (plus a lot more) at snack time. At the office, Diane couldn't usually resist when everyone took a break around 3:00 or 4:00 P.M. and raided the candy machines downstairs. Then after supper, she often rewarded herself with cookies ("They were low-fat!") when she did the laundry or paid the bills.

We went over her food diary. Lots of pasta, lots of sandwiches, potato chips, occasional chicken, occasional candy. Soft drinks almost daily. I asked her about red meat: She didn't much care for it, and as for trying to get her kids to eat it, fuggedaboudit.

Her biggest complaint about dieting? Hunger. Usually she dieted by eating only meals and cutting out the snacks, but she noticed that a couple of hours after every meal she'd be famished. One thousand calories, she'd tell herself. She watched the clock for lunchtime and was the first one out the door at 5:30, her stomach growling its complaints.

These last few years, every diet ended in disaster. She would lose weight, but after a few weeks the constant hunger and sense of deprivation would wear her down, and she would find herself gorging on any cookie or chip or candy she could find.

The other thing she hated about dieting was never eating

enough to really feel full. She measured out her portions oh-so-carefully, but a cup of pasta, wow, it sure didn't look like 250 calories. She liked to limit her meal calories so that she could treat herself with sweets for dessert. Without dessert, she felt she could never stick to a diet, because she would just feel even more deprived. She'd carefully measure out her ⅓ cup of ice cream (110 calories), savoring every spoonful. Filled with a feeling of real accomplishment, she could put the box away even when she was dying for more. But it never lasted.

"I just don't have the willpower."

After our talks and looking over her food diary and questionnaire, I thought Diane would do best on a fat-counting diet. What was it that made her a good candidate? First of all, her food preferences led her there. She ate lots of pasta, breads, and veggies. She rarely ate meat, and when she did, it was chicken or occasionally fish. What kept her from having a true low-fat diet were her high-fat snacks. Eating what she thought was a healthy low-calorie diet was making her hungry, and when she was hungry, the yummy treats of her officemates or in her cupboard were too hard to resist.

Even after a meal, she felt that she hadn't really eaten "enough." She wasn't really hungry, but she didn't feel really satisfied either. Eating a little of this and a little of that—the essence of a low-calorie diet—seemed silly, and she'd rather sit down to a huge salad than to a plate dotted with small servings of lots of different foods.

So what makes *you* a good low-fat dieter? Like Diane, you need to like the foods that make up a low-fat diet. So carbohydrates are going to play an important role: breads and pastas, fruits and vegetables; these foods make up the cornerstone of a fat-counting diet. You should be on this diet only if you love them. Low-fat proteins will also play an important role. This includes not only low-fat meats such as poultry and fish but also nonmeat sources of protein: beans, soy, dairy products, and eggs.

## WHO SHOULDN'T EAT A LOW-FAT DIET?

You probably shouldn't be on this diet if you have:

- Diabetes
- Metabolic syndrome
- High triglycerides
- Low HDL (good) cholesterol

These conditions suggest that you don't process carbohydrates normally, and carbs are the heart of this diet.

How you get full will also contribute to whether or not you do well on a low-fat diet. Volume should be an important satisfaction signal for successful low-fat dieters. It may seem obvious that, of course, everyone needs to have that feeling of fullness in her stomach to stop eating—but that's not true. We all have a variety of cues that tell us we've had enough. If you are reading this chapter, chances are you get your strongest sense of fullness from volume.

Although food preference and satisfaction are the two most important characteristics in choosing a low-fat diet, other aspects of your health and lifestyle also contribute. The presence of certain cardiac risk factors may have been key in selecting this type of diet for you.

And this diet requires you to eat frequently. Eating three meals per day plus two snacks will be essential for the maintenance of this diet. The snacks are as important as the meals. Why? Because for many eaters, and especially low-fat eaters, it's better to graze throughout the day, to ward off big hunger attacks. Those notorious collapses in the low-fat diet—those moments when you just can't take it anymore and you just have to dive headfirst into a bag of chocolate chip cookies until it's empty—are the problem. So you have to be willing to eat when you are hungry to enjoy this diet and make it work.

## THE BASICS OF A FAT-COUNTING DIET: MORE IS MORE

Fat contains more calories than any other form of food. The purpose of fat in our bodies—and in the bodies of the plants and animals that provide us with our fat—is to store energy. And it does that very well. A gram of carbohydrates or protein contains 4 calories. A gram of fat contains 9 calories—more than twice as many. That difference lies at the heart of the fat-counting diet.

Ultimately, a low-fat diet must be a low-calorie diet for you to lose weight. If you reduce the fat in your diet, while eating the right carbohydrates and proteins, you really can eat more food while taking in fewer calories. This works because of something we are reminded of every Thanksgiving. One of the most important ways we have of being satisfied by a meal is volume. In very concrete ways, in our stomachs, more is just, well, more. While we have ways of monitoring calories so that we end up eating the same number of calories on a day-to-day, week-to-week basis, our ability to figure the calories in a single meal is remarkably poor. We don't stop eating because we have taken in enough calories. In fact, when we stop eating, most of those calories are lying untouched in our stomachs.

What makes us stop is volume. And, in fact, most people eat the same volume of food each day. When researchers have done studies of men and women to see what triggers they have to make them stop eating, volume repeatedly comes out first. In other words, if you eat something that takes up a lot of room in your stomach but doesn't have very many calories, you are going to be more satisfied than if you ate something that didn't take up much room but had lots of calories.

Unfortunately, quantity may fool our stomachs on a single-meal basis—which is how most of these studies are done—but it doesn't always get us from one meal to the next. Eating a head of lettuce will fill you up, but chances are that in an hour or so you will be ready to eat again. Fats (and proteins) play an important role in keeping us feeling full so that we can last more than an hour or two between meals. You have to outsmart your body by keeping some fats and re-placing the rest with foods that have fewer calories but can send the same type of powerful message to the brain that you have eaten and that it was good.

## JOHN'S STORY

John is a 39-year-old Italian man who started and now runs a family-owned business. He was in pretty good shape when he was younger but began putting on weight after he had a family and started his business. By the time I met John, he was almost 50 pounds over what he considered to be his best weight. He had high blood pressure, and his knees hurt. He also had sleep apnea and needed to use a special air pump when he went to sleep every night. His cholesterol was out of control. His doctor told him that he would have to start taking medicine if he didn't get his LDL cholesterol levels down. He didn't want to take any medicines, but his father had had a heart attack in his fifties and John didn't want that either. That's when he came to see me.

John's days were hectic. He opened the shop at 7:30 each morn-ing and often didn't get home until after 9:00 P.M. When he got up in the mornings, he'd jump into the shower and rush off to work. He reported that he usually ate only one meal a day, dinner, because that was really the only meal he was hungry for. He never ate breakfast. Not hungry and no time, he said. If he got a few hunger pangs late in the morning, there was always something to snack on around the of-fice. He rarely stopped for lunch. He might grab a slice of pizza or a bag of fries—whatever the kids in the shop were eating. By the time he sat down for dinner, he was starving. Sometimes he felt like he ate all night long, from the moment he got home until he went to bed, because he just couldn't get a feeling of really being full.

Like Diane, his diet was primarily carbohydrates. He did eat meat, but usually fish or chicken, and he rarely had milk or butter. Cheese was a staple only because it came with the pizza he ate at the office.

John had been on a diet several years ago. He'd joined Weight Watchers and had lost almost 50 pounds over the course of the year. He'd tried to put himself back on that diet but had never really gotten it to work for him. He couldn't stick to it, because he felt hungry all the time.

After reviewing John's history and questionnaire, it seemed clear to me that a fat-counting diet would be best for him. It was right for his taste and temperament, it was right for his health, and it had worked in the past. I thought that John was having trouble making it work because he was trying to cut out fats without changing the rest of his diet, and that simply didn't work. And when he wasn't dieting, his habit of eating only one meal a day was contributing to the problem. By making him get so hungry that he couldn't keep himself from overeating, his eating habits were a big part of the problem.

John, like many dieters, allowed himself to starve all day long, and when he finally sat down to eat, he was driven to overeat. It's your body's natural reaction to deprivation, and it's as inevitable as gravity. No matter whether you are trying to lose weight or just maintain the weight you have, it's important that you eat when you are hungry, not when you are starving.

That is particularly important on a fat-counting diet. When you eat a diet high in carbohydrates, as you will on a fat-counting diet, you are providing your body with its preferred fuel. That means your body will be able to use these calories right away—and that's good. What that means, though, is that you will need to refuel at regular intervals to keep your body running. That means three meals a day and probably a snack or two. Otherwise, you end up too hungry once you are at the table and, like John, find yourself unable to stop.

## THE PERFECT FIT COUNTING FATS BASIC DIET

So what does a fat-counting diet look like? In this eating plan, probably more than any other, you have to think about not only the foods you're avoiding but also the foods you'll be replacing them with. Although the supermarket carries hundreds of low-fat products; many of them may not be low in calories.

On this diet, you will be eating some fat. And the fats you eat will be the "right" fats—those that are good for you. In addition, you'll be eating lots of naturally low-fat carbohydrates. You will be eating plenty of protein, because while carbs fill up your stomach, proteins help you feel satisfied and stay that way for hours at a time.

## THE SKINNY ON FAT

All fats are not created equal.

The Perfect Fit Counting Fats Diet provides you with about one-third of your calories from fat. This allows you some of the satisfying qualities of fat while reducing your total fat intake.

But it's not just a matter of getting rid of all kinds of fats. A healthy low-fat diet will eliminate the "bad" fats while increasing the "good" kind. Most of the fat in the average diet is bad: either saturated fats—those found in meat or high-fat dairy products—or a type known as trans fats. These are the fats that increase risk of heart disease and possibly cancer.

You may not have heard much about trans fats. They are only beginning to get the attention they deserve. These are found naturally

## THE HIDDEN COST OF LOW-FAT FOODS

Low-fat versions of foods frequently contain just as many calories—and sometimes even more—than their original version. In taking the fat out, manufacturers often put extra carbohydrates in. For example, low-fat peanut butter has one-third the amount of fat and yet still has 85 calories per tablespoon.

A regular oatmeal cookie made by one company has fewer calories than its fat-free version (45 calories versus 50). Read the label before you sample any low-fat foods to make sure they are low-calorie as well.

in tiny proportions in many foods, but most of the trans fats we eat are made in a laboratory (not that there's anything wrong with that). And though they fit the definition of monounsaturated or polyunsaturated fat, they act just like saturated fats in the body and seem to be linked to higher rates of coronary artery disease. Where do you find these trans-fatty acids? Wherever partially hydrogenated oils are sold. These are the fats used in many processed foods—cookies, breads, pastries. They add a creamy quality to the food and increase shelf life, so manufacturers love them. They also add to your risk of heart disease.

So, on the Counting Fats Diet, you reduce your intake of saturated fats by eating less meat and then only lean cuts of meat. And you will reduce trans fats by avoiding prepackaged baked goods and other foods containing these fats. Then you replace some of that fat with mono- and polyunsaturated fats—which are derived from nuts, grains, and olives—plus omega fats, which are found in seafood.

These healthful fats frequently make up only a small portion of the fat in a typical American diet. You can eat more of these and still get only 33 percent of your calories from fat. Because you need to

**HOW MUCH FAT?**

"No diet will remove all the fat from your body, because the brain is entirely fat. Without a brain, you might look good, but all you could do is run for public office." —GEORGE BERNARD SHAW

How much fat do you need in the diet? We all need some.

- Infants need to get 50 percent of their calories from fat.
- Children up to the age of 2 should get up to 40 percent of their calories from fat.
- Adults can get by with 15 to 20 percent of their calories from fat—if they want to.

make distinctions among fats, I don't call this a low-fat diet: I call it a fat-counting diet, because you pay attention not just to the fats you get rid of but to the fats you keep as well.

## THE SECRET OF THE COUNTING FATS DIET: KNOW YOUR LABELS

If you are going to reduce your fat to one-third of the calories in your diet and make sure you eat mostly "good" fats, you need to know how to read a food label. Sounds easy, but it can be confusing. The labeling of foods was the result of the pro-consumer movement that emerged in the 1970s, but the food industry managed to influence how the labels were written. So, yes, the information is there, but it's often there in surprisingly deceptive ways, ways meant to trick us into eating (and therefore buying) more.

First, you have to learn the lingo. Some foods say they are fat-free, and by law they can contain only 0.5 gram of fat or less per serving. Note that this is per serving. That's why you can have spray-on olive oil, and the label can claim that the product has no fat.

## HOW TO READ A LABEL

Check the calories per serving—you may be surprised at what you read. Saturated fat should make up less than 7 percent of your daily calories. On a 1,200-calorie diet, that's just 9 grams.

You should always check the serving size—all the information on the label is per serving. What you consider a serving may not match the USDA's idea of a serving.

Here's where the math comes in. To figure out the percentage of calories from fat, divide the total calories by the calories from fat. In this case, 90 ÷ 30 = 3. If your answer is less than 3, the food contains too much fat.

These numbers reflect how much of each nutrient is contained in a serving as a percent of the recommended daily allowance for a 2,000-calorie diet.

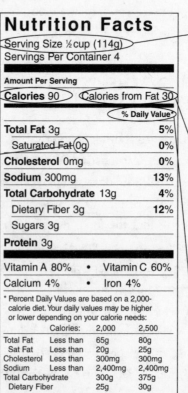

*Check the calories per serving—you may be surprised at what you read.*

*Saturated fat should make up less than 7 percent of your daily calories. On a 1,200-calorie diet, that's just 9 grams.*

*You should always check the serving size—all the information on the label is per serving. What you consider a serving may not match the USDA's idea of a serving.*

*Here's where the math comes in. To figure out the percentage of calories from fat, divide the total calories by the calories from fat. In this case, 90 ÷ 30 = 3. If your answer is less than 3, the food contains too much fat.*

*These numbers reflect how much of each nutrient is contained in a serving as a percent of the recommended daily allowance for a 2,000-calorie diet.*

### Nutrition Facts

Serving Size ½ cup (114g)
Servings Per Container 4

**Amount Per Serving**

**Calories** 90    Calories from Fat 30

% Daily Value*

| | |
|---|---|
| **Total Fat** 3g | **5%** |
| Saturated Fat 0g | **0%** |
| **Cholesterol** 0mg | **0%** |
| **Sodium** 300mg | **13%** |
| **Total Carbohydrate** 13g | **4%** |
| Dietary Fiber 3g | **12%** |
| Sugars 3g | |
| **Protein** 3g | |

| | | | |
|---|---|---|---|
| Vitamin A 80% | • | Vitamin C 60% | |
| Calcium 4% | • | Iron 4% | |

* Percent Daily Values are based on a 2,000-calorie diet. Your daily values may be higher or lower depending on your calorie needs:

| | | Calories: | 2,000 | 2,500 |
|---|---|---|---|---|
| Total Fat | Less than | | 65g | 80g |
| Sat Fat | Less than | | 20g | 25g |
| Cholesterol | Less than | | 300mg | 300mg |
| Sodium | Less than | | 2,400mg | 2,400mg |
| Total Carbohydrate | | | 300g | 375g |
| Dietary Fiber | | | 25g | 30g |

Calories per gram:

The amount you spray will contain less than 0.5 gram of fat. "Low-fat" means that each serving contains less than 3 grams of fat. "Reduced-fat" means that the product has 25 percent less fat than the original product. That's why you can have reduced-fat butter. It's not low-fat, but it has less fat.

The label will also tell you how many calories are in each serving. Knowledge is power: You need to know how many calories a food has, because it can really surprise you.

The label tells you what a serving is. Often what you think of as a single serving might not be what is listed as a serving on the label. Take a 20-ounce bottle of soda that comes out of a soda machine. You might think that's just one large serving—but you'd be wrong. That 20-ounce bottle contains "2.5 servings." The calorie count on the side tells you how many calories are in what the company calls a "portion." So there aren't 200 calories in that bottle of blue Gatorade; there are actually 500 calories. If you didn't read the servings per bottle info on the label, you'd never know that.

The food label will also tell you how much fat is in each serving, and it will list how much of that fat is saturated fat. You want to limit regular fats on this diet to 33 percent, and you want to limit saturated fats to less than 7 percent of your total caloric intake.

Here's what's not on the label: What percentage of the calories in the food comes from fat. For that you have to do a little math: Divide the number of calories in the serving by the number of calories from fat. If that number is less than 3, then more than a third of the calories come from fat, and you want to limit how much of that food you eat.

Here's another thing not on the label: How much of the fat is monounsaturated and polyunsaturated fat? You might think you could figure that out simply by subtracting the saturated fats from the total fat and you would end up with the amount of mono- and polyunsaturated fats. But you wouldn't, because manufacturers don't have to list the trans fats. At least not yet. The FDA has passed a rule, though, that they have to be listed as of January 2006. Until then, you can look on the panel listing the ingredients, and if you see the phrase "partially hydrogenated oils," then you know trans fats are in the food, though you won't know the amount.

Now, if you're not eating fats, what are you eating? A diet that restricts fats can work only if you make sure the carbohydrates and proteins that you eat will take over the job of making you feel full with fewer calories.

## THE RIGHT STUFF: PROTEIN

Proteins are the backbone of any successful diet. First of all, they are foods that help make you feel full. Carbohydrates alone can't do it. If you neglect your protein, you will feel hungry, and if you feel hungry, you will not be able to maintain your diet. What this means is that every meal and every snack should contain at least a small amount of protein to keep you feeling satisfied and full.

Second, your body needs protein every day because body parts (made primarily of protein) have to be repaired, and you have virtually no storage capacity for proteins. So you need to eat proteins every day. When you are restricting calories, your body will turn to muscle for the extra calories to keep running, often before it looks to fat stores. You don't want to lose muscle mass when you lose weight, because muscle helps burn calories. So what's a dieter to do? Eat more protein, say the studies.

Meat is the richest source of protein. Each ounce of beef contains 9 to 10 grams of protein. But it's also the form highest in fat—mostly saturated fat. So, on this diet you should look to nonmeat sources of protein for much of each day's supply. Dairy products have protein in them: Each cup of low-fat milk or yogurt contains 8 grams of protein; each ounce of low-fat cheese has 7 to 8 grams. Starchy beans (like navy beans or pinto beans, not the green beans you snap) have about 10 grams per cup. How much protein you'll be needing when you are dieting is based on your weight. In general, you should eat about 5 grams of protein for every 20 pounds of your current weight. You should try to get your protein from all the different classes of foods on a low-fat diet.

For example, a 150-pound woman should eat 35 grams of protein each day. She'd get that with 2 cups of 1% milk (remember, it goes in your coffee and your cereal), a container of low-fat yogurt or cottage cheese, a cup of three-bean salad, a string cheese stick, and 3 ounces of lean meat. A 200-pound man would get enough protein with 2 cups of low-fat milk, a poached egg, a slice of Canadian bacon, a container of yogurt, a handful of nuts, 4 ounces of fish, a serving of rice and beans, and a scoop of frozen yogurt. That's a lot of food.

I don't want you to feel as if you have to go around counting your protein. It's hard enough just keeping track of the fat. But I do want you to get an idea of just how much protein we need to keep our bodies running well and our bellies full.

## THE RIGHT STUFF: CARBOHYDRATES

Carbohydrates will continue to make up the largest category of foods you eat on a fat-counting diet. Like meat, carbohydrates can come attached to large amounts of fat. This is especially true of carbs you don't prepare yourself. Fats are often added to packaged foods in order to beef up the taste and lengthen shelf life. On this diet, you need to avoid prepackaged foods and go back to basics. This means not buying frozen meals or canned or frozen prepared foods. You might be thinking, Oh, I just don't have time for that! I understand, but many of the foods that make up a fat-counting diet don't take any longer to prepare than microwavable TV dinners, they are better tasting, and let's face it, much better for you.

The carbohydrates you eat on the Perfect Fit Counting Fats Diet, like the fats you eat, need to be the right variety. Some carbohydrates will make you feel full and satisfied. Others will leave you craving more—if not right away then in an hour or two. How can you distinguish between the right carbs and the wrong ones? Researchers have come up with a system to help you do just that called the glycemic load. Foods with a low GL will help you feel full, while

## 10 TIPS TO REDUCE YOUR FAT INTAKE

1. Limit your total fat intake to one-third of your total calories consumed in a day.

   • On a 1,500-calorie diet, this means 55 grams of fat.

   • On a 1,200-calorie diet, this means 44 grams of fat.

2. Limit your saturated fat intake to less than 7 percent of your total calorie intake in a day.

   • On a 1,500-calorie diet, this means only 12 grams of saturated fat.

   • On a 1,200-calorie diet, this means only 9 grams of saturated fat.

3. To do this…

   • Limit red meat, such as beef, to one or two meals per week, and when you eat it, cut off visible fat.

   • Avoid ground meats—even those marked "extra lean" contain more fat than a T-bone steak.

   • Remove the skin from poultry.

   • Roast, broil, or bake when you can.

   • If you need to cook in fat, sauté in olive oil.

   • Limit portions to 3 to 4 ounces at each meal (palm-size servings).

   • Avoid ready-prepared foods.

4. Limit butter and avoid margarine altogether. Margarine doesn't taste as good as butter and, because of the trans-fatty acids, is just as bad for you. (There are some buttery spreads with no trans fats.)

those with a high GL will make you feel hungry. (For more on glycemic load and for a list of common foods and their glycemic loads, see page 124.)

Generally, low-GL foods include fruits, vegetables, and foods made from whole grains. These are what many people call "whole

5. Use only 1% or fat-free milk and low-fat or fat-free cheeses.

6. Eat seafood as often as you can. It does have fat (though usually much less than beef), but it has little saturated fat and is loaded with omega fatty acids, which still have lots of calories, but can reduce your risk of heart disease.

7. Plan your meals around a carbohydrate and use the fat-containing foods as a flavor ingredient rather than as the focus of the meal.

8. When you eat eggs, use fewer yolks than whites. The yolks contain all the cholesterol, and a 2:3 or even 2:4 ratio of egg yolks to egg whites is just as flavorful with much less fat and cholesterol.

9. Replace high-fat foods with low-glycemic-load carbohydrates plus some protein whenever possible. Instead of snacking on a bag of chips, eat a piece of fruit or vegetable with a low-fat cheese or yogurt, or dip your veggies in hummus.

10. Eat vegetarian for one or two meals per week. Vegetarian cuisine is filled with foods that make you feel full while limiting fat intake. Vegetarian meals use a wide variety of beans and grains to provide the protein and low-glycemic-load carbohydrates that make up a healthy and satisfying low-fat diet.

11. (An extra) Try different seasonings. Fat is an easy way to add flavor to foods, but there are many sauces and flavoring strategies that can provide just as much flavor with virtually no fat. (I've given some ideas for flavoring low-fat meats, seafood, and vegetables in the recipe section at the end of this chapter.)

foods," that is, foods that have not been processed—foods we eat pretty much as they come. High-GL foods are usually foods that have been refined. Think of foods made from white flour, like breads, cookies, and pastries. Can this make weight loss easier? Research says yes: Eating a diet packed with low-GL foods has been shown to help people lose weight at least in part by making them feel full for longer.

Does the Counting Fats Diet work? It does for people who like to eat this way. Let's go back to Diane. She started a low-fat, low-glycemic-load diet and went from 205 to 180 in 4 months. As hard as it was, she made a point of eating breakfast with her kids every day. And she started bringing in her lunch every day to work. She was worried that she would feel left out when the other women went to the corner deli, but most of them started bringing in their lunches, too. It gives them a lot more time to sit and talk. She also began exercising every day. She told me that she'd never before felt so good. She's continued to lose weight, although not nearly as quickly. She now weighs 170. She's still not at her target, but she's getting there. Her sister was so intrigued by Diane's success that she started on the diet as well. Now they are exercising together every day.

And what about John? It was tough initially, but he's eating three meals a day, and just doing that has made him feel a lot better. The office is still filled with the kind of food he doesn't want to eat despite his attempt to ban them. He brings in his own snacks, however, and that goes a long way toward keeping him satisfied so that most days he can walk past the pizza without stopping. He lost 20 pounds in his first 3 months on his diet and has gone back to practicing his tae kwon do almost every day. His blood pressure is down and so is his cholesterol.

What does a low-fat, low-glycemic-load diet look like? To help you put these theories into practice, I have provided a list of foods in quantities that contain 5 grams of fat or less, a 7-day meal plan, and some tasty low-fat recipes.

# THE PERFECT FIT COUNTING FATS DIET: THE BIG PICTURE

- Reduce total fat to 33 percent of your calories.

- Eat the right fats by avoiding saturated and trans fats while enjoying mono- and polyunsaturated fats and omega fats.

- Eat the right carbohydrates by replacing processed, high-glycemic-load foods with whole, low-glycemic-load carbs.

- Include a low-fat protein in every meal and snack to help you feel full longer.

## FOOD LIST FOR COUNTING FATS BASIC DIET

These low-fat foods in the amounts listed contain 5 grams of fat or less. (Calories for portion sizes are also included. These are based on typical single-serving sizes.)

| FOOD | AMOUNT | CALORIES |
| --- | --- | --- |
| **VEGETABLES** | | |
| Artichoke | Unlimited | 60 per globe |
| Asparagus | Unlimited | 36 per 10 spears |
| Avocado | ⅙ fruit | 51 per ⅙ fruit |
| Beans, baked | 6 oz | 200 per 6 oz |
| Beans, black | Unlimited | 90 per ½ cup |
| Beans, kidney | Unlimited | 105 per ½ cup |
| Beans, lima | Unlimited | 100 per ½ cup |
| Beets | Unlimited | 44 per ½ cup |
| Black-eyed peas | 5 cups | 100 per ½ cup |
| Broccoli | Unlimited | 22 per ½ cup |
| Brussels sprouts | 4 cups | 302 per ½ cup |
| Cabbage | Unlimited | 17 per ½ cup |
| Carrots | Unlimited | 31 per large carrot |

| | | |
|---|---|---|
| Cauliflower | Unlimited | 25 per 1 cup |
| Celery | Unlimited | 20 per 1 cup |
| Chickpeas | 2½ cups | 100 per 1 cup |
| Corn on the cob | 3 ears | 123 per large ear |
| Cucumbers | 8 whole | 34 per cucumber |
| Eggplant | Unlimited | 28 per 1 cup cubed |
| Lettuce (all varieties) | Unlimited | 7 per 1 cup |
| Mushrooms | Unlimited | 5 per mushroom |
| Onion | Unlimited | 29 per ½ cup |
| Peas, green | Unlimited | 60 per ½ cup |
| Peppers, bell, fresh | 5 medium | 25 per large fruit |
| Potato | Unlimited | 220 per large potato |
| Potato, sweet | Unlimited | 185 per large potato |
| Radishes | Unlimited | 2 per large radish |
| Soybeans (edamame) | ⅓ cup | 98 per ⅓ cup |
| Spinach | Unlimited | 81 per 1 cup |
| Squash, summer | Unlimited | 36 per 1 cup |
| Squash, winter | Unlimited | 80 per 1 cup |
| Tomato, canned | Unlimited | 25 per ½ cup |
| Tomato, fresh | Unlimited | 38 per large fruit |
| Yam | Unlimited | 158 per 1 cup |
| Zucchini | 10 large | 45 per fruit |

## FRUITS

| | | |
|---|---|---|
| Apples | Unlimited | 81 per fruit |
| Apricots | Unlimited | 17 per fruit |
| Bananas | 7 large | 140 per fruit |
| Blueberries | 5 pints | 225 per pint/38 per 50 berries |
| Cantaloupe | Unlimited | 72 per ¼ fruit |
| Cherries | Unlimited | 52 per 1 cup |
| Coconut | ½ ounce | 67 per ½ oz |
| Grapefruit | Unlimited | 46 per ½ fruit |
| Grapes | 10 cups | 57 per ½ cup/approx. 14 grapes |

| Kiwifruit | 8 fruits | 56 per large fruit |
|---|---|---|
| Mango | 8 fruits | 135 per large fruit |
| Olives | 5 medium | 46 per 5 medium olives |
| Oranges | 10 medium | 86 per large fruit |
| Pears | 7 medium | 123 per large fruit |
| Plums | 7 large | 36 per fruit |
| Prunes | Unlimited | 20 per large fruit |
| Raisins | Unlimited | 130 per ¼ cup |
| Raspberries | Unlimited | 153 per pint |
| Strawberries | Unlimited | 46 per 1 cup |
| Watermelon | 7 cups | 49 per 1 cup |

## MEAT, POULTRY, AND SEAFOOD (All meats are trimmed of visible fat.)

### BEEF

| Beef brisket | 1 oz | 179 per 3 oz |
|---|---|---|
| Beef loin | 2½ oz | 168 per 3 oz |
| Chuck & pot roast | 6 oz | 179 per 3 oz |
| Flank steak | 2 oz | 176 per 3 oz |
| Sirloin | 2½ oz | 162 per 3 oz |
| Top round | 3 oz | 169 per 3 oz |

### LAMB

| Lamb chop | ½ oz | 200 per 3 oz |
|---|---|---|
| Leg of lamb | 3 oz | 140 per 3 oz |

### PORK

| Bacon | 1½ slices | 109 per 3 slices |
|---|---|---|
| Bacon, Canadian style | 3 slices | 86 per 2 slices |
| Ham | 3 oz | 133 per 3 oz |
| Pepperoni | 2 slices | 27 per slice |
| Pork chop | 2 oz | 182 per 3 oz |
| Pork loin | 3 oz | 199 per 3 oz |
| Pork sausage | ½ link | 100 per link |

## POULTRY

| | | |
|---|---|---|
| Chicken, dark, no skin | 1½ oz | 232 per 4 oz |
| Chicken, white, no skin | 4 oz | 187 per 4 oz |
| Turkey, dark, no skin | 3 oz | 212 per 4 oz |
| Turkey, white, no skin | 6 oz | 178 per 4 oz |
| Turkey sausage | 2 links | 46 per link |

## SEAFOOD

| | | |
|---|---|---|
| Clams | 11 oz | 133 per 3 oz |
| Cod, Atlantic | Unlimited | 89 per 3 oz |
| Crabs | 11 oz | 84 per 3 oz |
| Flounder | 16 oz | 99 per 3 oz |
| Haddock | 12 oz | 95 per 3 oz |
| Lobster | 20 oz | 142 per 4 oz |
| Mussels | 4 oz | 146 per 3 oz |
| Oysters | 9 oz | 61 per 3 oz |
| Salmon, canned | 12 oz | 120 per 3 oz |
| Salmon, fresh farmed | 1½ oz | 175 per 3 oz |
| Shrimp, medium | 15 oz/approx. 60 shrimp | 100 per 4 oz |
| Swordfish | 3 oz | 132 per 3 oz |
| Trout | 2 oz | 162 per 3 oz |
| Tuna, in water | 7 oz | 99 per 3 oz |
| Tuna, fresh | 12 oz | 112 per 3 oz |

## CHEESE

| | | |
|---|---|---|
| American, light | 1⅓ slices | 55 per slice |
| Cheddar, low-fat | 2½ oz | 49 per 1 oz |
| Cottage cheese | ½ cup | 120 per ½ cup |
| Cottage cheese, 1% | 5 cups | 90 per ½ cup |
| Cream cheese, lite | 1 oz | 60 per 1 oz |
| Feta | ¾ oz | 75 per 1 oz |
| Mozzarella, part-skim | 1 oz | 72 per 1 oz |
| Parmesan | ⅔ oz | 129 per 1 oz |
| Ricotta, part-skim | 2 oz | 39 per 1 oz |

| String cheese | 1 oz | 80 per 1 oz |
| Swiss, low-fat | 1 oz | 90 per 1 oz |

## DAIRY

| | | |
|---|---|---|
| Cream, half-and-half | ⅓ cup | 315 per 1 cup |
| Egg, cooked omelet style | ½ egg | 93 per egg |
| Egg, hard-boiled | ¾ egg | 78 per egg |
| Egg white from 1 egg | Unlimited | 17 per egg |
| Egg yolk from 1 egg | 1 egg | 59 per egg |
| Frozen yogurt, fat-free | Unlimited | 100 per ½ cup |
| Ice cream, vanilla | ¼ cup | 140 per ½ cup |
| Ice cream, vanilla, fat-free | Unlimited | 100 per ½ cup |
| Ice cream sandwich | ¼ bar | 170 per bar |
| Milk, fat-free | 5 cups | 90 per cup |
| Milk, 2% | 1½ cups | 130 per 1 cup |
| Milk, whole | ⅔ cup | 157 per 1 cup |
| Sour cream | 2 tbsp | 26 per 1 tbsp |
| Sour cream, fat-free | Unlimited | 30 per 1 tbsp |
| Yogurt, fat-free | Unlimited | 100 per 1 cup |
| Yogurt, low-fat, fruit-flavored | 1½ cups | 240 per 1 cup |
| Yogurt, low-fat, plain | 1 cup | 140 per 1 cup |

## FATS AND OILS

| | | |
|---|---|---|
| Butter | ¾ tbsp | 55 per 1 tbsp |
| Hummus | 1½ tbsp | 25 per 1 tbsp |
| Margarine | 1½ tbsp | 34 per 1 tbsp |
| Margarine, light | 5 tbsp | 50 per 1 tbsp |
| Margarine, low-fat | 5 tbsp | 25 per 1 tbsp |
| Mayonnaise | ½ tbsp | 100 per 1 tbsp |
| Mayonnaise, light | 1 tbsp | 50 per 1 tbsp |
| Mayonnaise, low-fat | 5 tbsp | 25 per 1 tbsp |
| Olive oil | 1 tsp | 119 per 1 tbsp |
| Vegetable oil | 1 tsp | 120 per 1 tbsp |

## NUTS AND SEEDS

| | | |
|---|---|---|
| Almonds | ⅓ oz/approx. 9 nuts | 164 per 1 oz |
| Brazil nuts | ⅓ oz/approx. 2 nuts | 186 per 1 oz |
| Cashews | ⅓ oz | 180 per 1 oz |
| Macadamia nuts | 2 nuts | 204 per 1 oz/10 nuts |
| Pecans | ¼ oz | 196 per 1 oz |
| Pine nuts | ⅓ oz/approx. 50 nuts | 160 per 1 oz |
| Pistachio nuts | ⅓ oz/approx. 15 nuts | 156 per 1 oz |
| Sunflower seeds | ⅓ cup/approx. 50 seeds | 160 per 1 oz |
| Walnuts | ⅙ cup/approx. 4 halves | 180 per ½ cup |

## BREADS, GRAINS, AND PASTA

| | | |
|---|---|---|
| Bread, light | Unlimited | 40 per slice |
| Bread (most varieties) | 5 slices | 80 per slice |
| English muffin | Unlimited | 140 per muffin |
| Pasta | 10 oz (5 cups) | 210 per ½ cup |
| Popcorn | 2½ cups | 100 per 3 cups |
| Popcorn, light | 7 cups | 60 per 3 cups |
| Rice, brown | 2½ cups (cooked) | 216 per 1 cup |
| Rice, white | 5 cups (cooked) | 205 per 1 cup |
| Rice, wild | Unlimited | 163 per 1 cup |
| Rice cake, cheese | 2½ cups | 60 per cake |
| Rice cake, plain | 10 cups | 60 per cake |
| Taco shells | 1 shell | 98 per shell |
| Wheat germ | 2 oz | 108 per 1 oz |

## CEREALS

| | | |
|---|---|---|
| All-Bran | 5 cups | 79 per ½ cup |
| Cream of wheat | Unlimited | 116 per ¾ cup |
| Fiber One | 6 cups | 62 per ½ cup |
| Oatmeal | 2½ cups | 99 per ¾ cup |
| Raisin bran | Unlimited | 178 per 1 cup |

## COOKIES AND CRACKERS

| | | |
|---|---|---|
| Animal crackers | 15 cookies | 141 per 12 cookies |
| Chips Ahoy chocolate chip cookies | 1½ cookies | 68 per 1 cookie |
| Melba toast | Unlimited | 16 per cracker |
| Wheatables | 15 crackers | 70 per 12 crackers |
| Wheat Thins | 15 crackers | 140 per 16 crackers |

## BEVERAGES

| | | |
|---|---|---|
| Coca-Cola | Unlimited | 145 per 12 oz |
| Coffee | Unlimited | 5 per 1 cup |
| Diet Coke | Unlimited | 2 per 12 oz |
| Juices | Unlimited | 100 per 1 cup |
| Root beer | Unlimited | 152 per 12 oz |
| Soy milk | 1 cup | 81 per 1 cup |

# DAILY MEAL PLANS FOR THE COUNTING FATS DIET

(Recipes for dishes in **bold print** are listed alphabetically in the recipe section at the end of the chapter on page 216.)

## DAY 1

| | Fat (g) | Calories |
|---|---|---|
| **Breakfast** | | |
| 1 cup high-fiber cereal (Bran Flakes or 100% Bran) | 2 | 120 |
| ½ cup 1% or ¾ cup fat-free milk | 1 | 45 |
| ½ cup fresh berries | 0 | 40 |
| 1 slice low-calorie, high-fiber bread | 1 | 40 |
| 1 tablespoon peanut butter | 8 | 95 |
| Total fat and calories | 12 | 340 |
| **A.M. Snack** | | |
| 2 tablespoons hummus | 3 | 50 |
| Sliced celery and carrots | 0 | 50 |
| Total fat and calories | 3 | 100 |
| **Lunch** | | |
| 1 cup black bean soup | 1.5 | 115 |
| 1 ripe tomato, sliced | 0 | 25 |
| 1 ounce reduced-fat mozzarella cheese, sliced | 4 | 70 |
| 2 tablespoons chopped fresh basil | 5 | 25 |
| Wasa crispbread, 2 crackers | 0 | 45 |
| Total fat and calories | 10.5 | 280 |
| **P.M. Snack** | | |
| 8 ounces fat-free yogurt | 0 | 100 |
| Total fat and calories | 0 | 100 |

### Dinner

| | Fat (g) | Calories |
|---|---|---|
| **Lemon Chicken Cutlets** | 11 | 355 |
| ½ cup brown rice | 1 | 110 |
| 1 cup broccoli, steamed and served with lemon | 0 | 45 |
| Total fat and calories | 12 | 510 |
| **Total fat and calories for Day 1** | **37.5** | **1,330** |

# DAY

| | Fat (g) | Calories |
|---|---|---|
| **Breakfast** | | |
| ½ cup oatmeal (not instant—the regular stuff cooks in 2–3 minutes in the microwave oven and has a much lower glycemic index) with ½ cup fat-free milk and 1 teaspoon sugar | 1 | 135 |
| ¼ cantaloupe | 0 | 70 |
| 1 slice low-calorie bread, toasted | 1 | 40 |
| 1 tablespoon low-fat peanut butter | 8 | 95 |
| Total fat and calories | 10 | 340 |
| **A.M. Snack** | | |
| String cheese stick | 5 | 80 |
| 1 medium apple | 0.5 | 80 |
| Total fat and calories | 5.5 | 160 |
| **Lunch** | | |
| **Black and White Bean Salad** | 4 | 175 |
| 10 reduced-fat Wheat Thins crackers | 2.5 | 85 |
| Total fat and calories | 6.5 | 260 |
| **P.M. Snack** | | |
| FrozFruit bar | 0.5 | 60 |
| Total fat and calories | 0.5 | 60 |

### Dinner

| | Fat (g) | Calories |
|---|---|---|
| **Chicken Pot Pie** | 7 | 305 |
| Romaine lettuce, tomatoes, and artichoke hearts | 1 | 100 |
| **Vinaigrette** | 5 | 35 |
| ½ cup strawberries | 0.5 | 50 |
| 2 tablespoons Cool Whip | 1 | 25 |
| Total fat and calories | 14.5 | 515 |
| **Total fat and calories for Day 2** | **37** | **1,335** |

# DAY 3

| | Fat (g) | Calories |
|---|---|---|
| **Breakfast** | | |
| 3-egg omelet using 2 yolks and 3 whites, filled with 1 cup chopped onion, green bell peppers, and tomato | 10 | 285 |
| ½ grapefruit with 1 teaspoon sugar | 0 | 60 |
| Total fat and calories | 10 | 345 |
| **A.M. Snack** | | |
| Grapes (approx. 2 dozen) | 0.5 | 80 |
| Total fat and calories | 0.5 | 80 |
| **Lunch** | | |
| 1 cup chicken vegetable soup | 1.5 | 90 |
| **Vegetable Sandwich** | 14.5 | 280 |
| Total fat and calories | 16 | 370 |
| **P.M. Snack** | | |
| 3 cups light popcorn | 1 | 60 |
| Total fat and calories | 1 | 60 |

### Dinner

| | Fat (g) | Calories |
|---|---|---|
| 1 serving **Pork Chops with Sweet Potatoes and Apples** | 10 | 300 |
| 10 stalks asparagus steamed, seasoned with lemon | 0 | 36 |
| Small fresh salad with **Vinaigrette** | 5 | 100 |
| Total fat and calories | 15 | 436 |
| **Total fat and calories for Day 3** | **42.5** | **1,291** |

# DAY 4

|  | Fat (g) | Calories |
|---|---|---|
| **Breakfast** | | |
| 1 cup high-fiber cereal (Bran Flakes or 100% Bran) | 2 | 120 |
| ½ cup 1% or ¾ cup fat-free milk | 1 | 45 |
| ½ cup fresh berries | 0 | 40 |
| 2 slices Canadian bacon | 4 | 90 |
| Total fat and calories | 7 | 295 |
| **A.M. Snack** | | |
| 16 reduced-fat Wheat Thins crackers | 4 | 120 |
| Total fat and calories | 4 | 120 |
| **Lunch** | | |
| Ham and Swiss cheese sandwich with lettuce and tomato on low-calorie bread with mustard | 12 | 255 |
| Carrot sticks | 0 | 50 |
| Total fat and calories | 12 | 305 |
| **P.M. Snack** | | |
| 1 large apple | 0 | 120 |
| Total fat and calories | 0 | 120 |

### Dinner

| | Fat (g) | Calories |
|---|---|---|
| 4-ounce tuna steak, broiled or grilled, topped with **Pico de Gallo** | 1.5 | 165 |
| 1 medium artichoke, steamed and dipped in **Vinaigrette** | 5 | 75 |
| ½ cup lima beans, steamed (frozen are great) | 0 | 85 |
| ½ cup frozen yogurt | 5 | 150 |
| Total fat and calories | 11.5 | 475 |
| **Total fat and calories for Day 4** | **34.5** | **1,315** |

# DAY 5

| | Fat (g) | Calories |
|---|---|---|
| **Breakfast** | | |
| **Fruit Smoothie** | 4 | 310 |
| 1 slice low-calorie bread, toasted | 1 | 40 |
| 2 tablespoons hummus | 3 | 50 |
| Total fat and calories | 8 | 400 |
| **A.M. Snack** | | |
| 1 cup cut celery, carrots, and broccoli | 0 | 50 |
| Total fat and calories | 0 | 50 |
| **Lunch** | | |
| **Greek Salad** | 12 | 175 |
| 1 small pita bread | 0.5 | 75 |
| Total fat and calories | 12.5 | 250 |
| **P.M. Snack** | | |
| Grapes (about 2 dozen) | 0.5 | 80 |
| Total fat and calories | 0.5 | 80 |

### Dinner

| | | |
|---|---|---|
| **Beef Stroganoff** | 15 | 395 |
| 1 cup broccoli | 0 | 45 |
| FrozFruit bar | 0.5 | 60 |
| Total fat and calories | 15.5 | 500 |

| | | |
|---|---|---|
| **Total fat and calories for Day 5** | **36.5** | **1,280** |

# DAY 6

| | Fat (g) | Calories |
|---|---|---|

### Breakfast

| | | |
|---|---|---|
| 3-egg omelet using 2 yolks and 3 whites, filled with chopped onion, green bell peppers, and tomato | 10 | 185 |
| 2 slices Canadian bacon, grilled or warmed in microwave oven | 4 | 90 |
| ½ grapefruit with 1 teaspoon sugar | 0 | 60 |
| Total fat and calories | 14 | 335 |

### A.M. Snack

| | | |
|---|---|---|
| 1 large pear | 0 | 125 |
| Total fat and calories | 0 | 125 |

### Lunch

| | | |
|---|---|---|
| 1 cup Manhattan clam chowder | 2 | 80 |
| Ham and Swiss cheese sandwich with lettuce and tomato on low-calorie bread with mustard | 12 | 240 |
| Total fat and calories | 14 | 320 |

### P.M. Snack

| | | |
|---|---|---|
| 3 cups popcorn | 1 | 60 |
| Total fat and calories | 1 | 60 |

### Dinner

| | Fat (g) | Calories |
|---|---|---|
| Boiled shrimp (about 16 large) | 2 | 100 |
| Cocktail sauce (ketchup and horseradish) | 3 | 60 |
| 1 ear corn on the cob (no butter) | 0 | 125 |
| 2 cups salad with 2 tablespoons **Green Goddess Dressing** | 0 | 90 |
| 1 light ice cream sandwich | 1 | 100 |
| Total fat and calories | 6 | 475 |
| **Total fat and calories for Day 6** | **35** | **1,315** |

# DAY 7

| | Fat (g) | Calories |
|---|---|---|
| **Breakfast** | | |
| **Eggs Carbonara** | 18 | 320 |
| ½ cantaloupe | 0 | 100 |
| Total fat and calories | 18 | 420 |
| **A.M. Snack** | | |
| 8 ounces fat-free yogurt | 0 | 100 |
| Total fat and calories | 0 | 100 |
| **Lunch** | | |
| **Tuna and Corn Salad** served on 2 cups lettuce dressed in **Vinaigrette** | 12 | 210 |
| 10 Wheat Thins crackers | 2.5 | 85 |
| Total fat and calories | 14.5 | 295 |
| **P.M. Snack** | | |
| FrozFruit bar | 0.5 | 60 |
| Total fat and calories | 0.5 | 60 |

## Dinner

| | | |
|---|---|---|
| **Ratatouille** | 15 | 215 |
| Grilled chicken breast (4 ounces) | 3 | 140 |
| 1 cup steamed pea pods (snow peas) | 0 | 40 |
| ½ cup strawberries topped with 2 tablespoons Cool Whip | 1.5 | 75 |
| Total fat and calories | 19.5 | 470 |
| **Total fat and calories for Day 7** | **52.5** | **1,345** |

# RECIPES FOR FAT COUNTERS

For your convenience, the recipes are listed in alphabetical order.

## BEEF STROGANOFF

4    tablespoons all-purpose flour
     Salt
     Ground black pepper
¾    pound flank steak, cut into strips
4    tablespoons olive oil
2    cloves garlic, crushed
1½   cups sliced onions
1½   cups sliced green bell peppers
1    cup sliced mushrooms
1    cup fat-free beef broth
½    cup fat-free sour cream
1    package (1 pound) noodles, cooked according to
     package directions

In a shallow bowl, mix 3 tablespoons of the flour with the salt and black pepper to taste and dredge the steak in the flour mixture. Heat the oil in a large skillet over medium-high heat. Add the steak and cook, stirring frequently, for about 5 minutes, or until brown. Add the garlic, onions, and bell peppers and cook for 2 minutes, stirring frequently. Add the mushrooms and cook for another 2 minutes, stirring frequently. Add the beef broth and bring the mixture to a boil. Cover, reduce heat, and simmer for 10 minutes.

Meanwhile, in a small bowl, mix the sour cream and the remaining flour. Stir until smooth, then add into the simmering mixture. Cook for about 2 minutes, stirring frequently, until the mixture is thickened. Serve over noodles.

MAKES 4 SERVINGS
PER SERVING: 15 G FAT, 395 CALORIES

## BLACK AND WHITE BEAN SALAD

1   can (14–19 ounces) black beans, rinsed and drained
1   can (14–19 ounces) cannellini beans, rinsed and drained
½   cup cider vinegar
1   tablespoon olive oil
1–2 cloves garlic, minced
½   teaspoon red pepper flakes
2   large ripe tomatoes
1   medium onion
1   green or red bell pepper
2   ribs celery
2   large carrots
½   cup parsley, chopped
12  pitted olives
    Salt
    Ground black pepper
    Romaine lettuce or fresh spinach

In a large bowl, combine the black beans, cannellini beans, vinegar, oil, garlic, and red pepper flakes. (I often simmer the beans for about 5 minutes before using them. I think it makes them easier to digest—if you know what I mean.) Mix and set aside as you chop the tomatoes, onion, bell pepper, celery, carrots, parsley, and olives. Mix the vegetables with the beans and add salt and black pepper to taste. Serve on a bed of romaine lettuce or fresh spinach.

MAKES 6 SERVINGS
PER SERVING: 4 G FAT, 175 CALORIES

Note: You can substitute white or brown rice for the cannellini beans.

## CHICKEN POT PIE

1   tablespoon olive oil
1   small onion, chopped

2　ribs celery, chopped

1　green bell pepper, chopped

1　cup sliced carrots

2　cups sliced fresh mushrooms

1　pound cooked chicken, cut into small pieces

1　cup frozen green peas (see note)

1　cup low-fat chicken broth

3　tablespoons flour

1　cup reduced-fat biscuit mix

½　cup 1% milk

Heat the oil in a large nonstick skillet over medium-high heat. Add the onion, celery, bell pepper, and carrots and cook, stirring frequently, until the vegetables begin to soften. Add the mushrooms and cook, stirring frequently, until soft. Add the chicken and peas and cook, stirring frequently, until warm. Pour into a 13 × 9-inch baking dish.

In a small bowl, whisk 3 tablespoons of the chicken broth with the flour to form a smooth paste. Add the remainder of the chicken broth and stir until thickened. Pour into the baking dish with the chicken and vegetables.

In a bowl, combine the biscuit mix and milk to make a soft dough. Drop the dough by heaping tablespoons onto the chicken mixture to form 10 biscuits. Bake at 400°F for 20 to 25 minutes, or until the biscuits are golden.

MAKES 5 SERVINGS
PER SERVING: 7 G FAT, 305 CALORIES

Note: Frozen green peas are almost as good as fresh and a lot handier.

## EGGS CARBONARA

1　teaspoon butter

3　egg whites

2　egg yolks

½　cup lean ham, diced

½　cup frozen peas, thawed

¼　cup Parmesan cheese

In a nonstick skillet, melt the butter. In a small bowl, beat together the egg whites and egg yolks. When very fluffy, pour into the skillet. Cook over low heat until the edges are firm.

Heat the ham in a microwave oven. Add the ham and peas to half of the eggs, and fold the other half over. Cook until the top is firm. Sprinkle with the cheese before serving.

MAKES 2 SERVINGS
PER SERVING: 18 G FAT, 320 CALORIES

## FRUIT SMOOTHIE

I add a little All-Bran to my smoothies—I love it; others don't. Try it and see.

1    cup 1% milk
¼    cup plain yogurt
1    large ripe banana or other soft fruit, such as canned peaches or fresh or frozen berries
2–3 ice cubes
1    tablespoon All-Bran cereal (optional)

In a blender, combine the milk, yogurt, banana or other fruit, ice cubes, and cereal, if desired. Blend until smooth.

MAKES 1 SERVING
PER SERVING: 4 G FAT, 310 CALORIES

## GREEK SALAD

SALAD
6    cups lettuce, washed and shredded, or half lettuce and half spinach
1    medium tomato, cut into wedges
½    small onion, thinly sliced
2    ounces low-fat feta cheese, crumbled
6    Greek olives, pitted

DRESSING

¼   cup red wine

1   tablespoon olive oil

1   tablespoon dried oregano

2   teaspoons lemon juice

1   teaspoon chopped fresh basil or ½ teaspoon dried basil

*To make the salad:* In a large bowl, combine the lettuce or lettuce-spinach mixture with the tomato, onion, cheese, and olives.

*To make the dressing:* In a small bowl, mix the wine, oil, oregano, lemon juice, and basil. Pour the dressing over the salad and toss to mix.

MAKES 2 SERVINGS
PER SERVING: 12 G FAT, 175 CALORIES

# GREEN GODDESS DRESSING

1   cup low-fat plain yogurt

2   tablespoons low-fat mayonnaise

2   teaspoons lemon juice

1   teaspoon vinegar

1   clove garlic, minced

2   tablespoons parsley

½   teaspoon yellow mustard

1   teaspoon chopped fresh tarragon or ½ teaspoon dried tarragon

In a small bowl, combine the yogurt, mayonnaise, lemon juice, vinegar, garlic, parsley, mustard, and tarragon. Mix well.

MAKES 8 SERVINGS
PER SERVING: 0 G FAT, 14 CALORIES

## LEMON CHICKEN CUTLETS

3   tablespoons flour
    Salt
    Ground black pepper
2   chicken breast cutlets
1   tablespoon olive oil
    Juice of 1 lemon
1   tablespoon capers
¼   cup white wine

In a shallow bowl, mix the flour with salt and pepper to taste. Dredge the chicken cutlets in the flour mixture.

Heat the oil in a nonstick skillet. Add the chicken and cook for about 5 minutes, turning it over to make sure it cooks through. Take the chicken from the skillet and set aside. In the same skillet, combine the lemon juice, capers, and wine. Simmer until the sauce has reduced by half, 8 to 10 minutes. Return the chicken to the skillet. Lower the heat and simmer together for 3 to 5 minutes.

MAKES 2 SERVINGS
PER SERVING: 11 G FAT, 355 CALORIES

## PICO DE GALLO

2   cups tomatoes, peeled, seeded, and coarsely chopped
1   cup scallions, minced
1   jalapeño chile pepper, finely chopped (wear plastic gloves when handling) or red pepper flakes
2   tablespoons lime juice
1   clove garlic, minced
    Salt
    Ground black pepper
¼   cup chopped fresh cilantro leaves

In a bowl, combine the tomatoes, scallions, chile pepper or desired amount of red pepper flakes, lime juice, and garlic. Add salt and black pepper to taste. Stir in the cilantro. Refrigerate for 1 hour before serving.

MAKES 6 SERVINGS
PER SERVING: 1 G FAT, 10 CALORIES

## PORK CHOPS WITH
## SWEET POTATOES AND APPLES

3   tablespoons all-purpose flour
    Salt
    Ground black pepper
2   pork chops, 3 ounces each
¼   cup diced onion
½–1 cup chicken broth
¼   cup apple cider
1   small sweet potato, sliced
1   apple, sliced

In a shallow bowl, mix the flour with the salt and pepper to taste and dredge the pork chops in the flour mixture.

Heat a large nonstick skillet sprayed with olive oil over medium-high heat. Add the pork chops and cook for about 2 minutes on each side, or until brown. Remove from the skillet and set aside.

In the same skillet, combine the onion and a small amount of the chicken broth. Cook until the onion is tender and translucent. Add the cider and the remaining chicken broth. Add the sweet potato, let simmer for 5 minutes, then add the apple and pork chops. Add more broth as needed. Cover, reduce heat, and simmer 5-10 minutes until the sweet potato and apple are tender.

MAKES 2 SERVINGS
PER SERVING: 10 G FAT, 300 CALORIES

## RATATOUILLE

2    large eggplants, cut into ½-inch-thick slices

4    red or yellow bell peppers, cut into strips

4    large ripe red tomatoes, cored, peeled, seeded, and cut into thick slices

2    large onions, thinly sliced

5    cloves garlic, coarsely chopped

½    teaspoon dried thyme

     Salt

     Ground black pepper

¼    cup virgin olive oil

In a 13 × 9-inch baking dish, layer half of the eggplants, bell peppers, tomatoes, and onions. Add the garlic and thyme. Add salt and black pepper to taste. Top with the other half of the vegetables. Drizzle the dish with the oil. Bake for 1 hour at 350°F. Serve immediately.

MAKES 4 SERVINGS
PER SERVING: 15 G FAT, 215 CALORIES

## TUNA AND CORN SALAD

This recipe tastes best with fresh corn. Cook it in a microwave oven for 2 to 3 minutes, then cut it off the cob. If using frozen corn, cook it in a microwave oven for 1 minute, then rinse with cold water.

1    cup corn, fresh or frozen, cooked; or canned, drained

1    can (6 ounces) water-packed tuna

3    ribs celery, chopped

½    onion, finely chopped

½    cup low-fat mayonnaise

     Pimientos

     Salt

     Ground black pepper

In a bowl, mix together the corn, tuna, celery, onion, and mayonnaise. Add the pimientos and salt and pepper to taste.

MAKES 4 SERVINGS
PER SERVING: 7 G FAT, 175 CALORIES

## VEGETABLE SANDWICH

2    slices low-calorie bread
½    very ripe avocado
¼    cucumber, peeled and sliced
½    tomato, sliced
¼    onion, very thinly sliced
¼    green bell pepper, sliced
1    handful bean sprouts
1    tablespoon Jerusalem artichoke relish (see note)

On 1 slice of the low-calorie bread, spread the flesh of the avocado. Layer with the cucumber, tomato, onion, and bell pepper. Add the bean sprouts and relish. Top with the second slice of bread.

MAKES 1 SERVING
PER SERVING: 14.5 G FAT, 280 CALORIES

Note: For the Jerusalem artichoke relish, you may substitute any vegetable relish you like or Pico de Gallo (page 221).

## VINAIGRETTE

¼    cup olive oil
⅓     wine vinegar (see note)
⅓    cup water
1–2 cloves garlic, minced
     Salt
     Ground black pepper

In a small bowl, mix the oil, vinegar, water, and garlic. Add salt and pepper to taste.

MAKES 12 SERVINGS (1 CUP)
PER SERVING: 5 G FAT, 35 CALORIES

Note: You can replace up to half of the vinegar with mustard; Dijon mustard works best.

# PART 4

# TAILORING YOUR PERFECT FIT DIET TO YOUR TASTES AND TO YOUR LIFE

O KAY. YOU'VE ALREADY done all the heavy lifting: You've kept an eating and exercise diary, and you've filled out the questionnaire. You've scored it and found out which basic diet works best for you. It's time to customize that diet based on what you know about yourself.

Part 4 is broken up into chapters that correspond to sections in the questionnaire. At the end of each section I've given you the page numbers within these chapters, so that you can find the information relevant to your dieting profile. These chapters will give you all the guidance you need to tailor your diet based on everything that you have learned about yourself and about nutrition.

The first chapter in part 4 (chapter 9) deals with the types of foods you prefer, with tips on how to work your favorite kinds of foods into your basic diet. Are you a Carnimore? Are you a VegeCarian? A Starch Stealer? A Sweets Eater? You will find out how to work with these preferences in your diet to achieve the weight you want.

Chapter 10 deals with your dieting history and what makes you feel full and satisfied. Are you someone who needs to eat a certain volume of food in order to feel full? Do you find yourself bored by the foods you are allowed to eat? Do you crave variety? Do you have a hard time feeling full if you haven't eaten something rich, like meat or another source of protein? These are all characteristics of the ways we feel full. Each of us has all three of these satiety mechanisms at work, but for many of us, one predominates. Which one is most important to you? Assessing how past diets have worked or not will help you determine which type of cues rules your system.

Chapter 11 evaluates how your medical history and that of your family may affect which diet is going to work best for you. Are you a binge eater? Do you have high blood pressure or diabetes? Do you smoke? Your diet should be based on food preferences and what makes you feel full, but how your body works is also an important factor. What good is a diet if it makes you feel worse because it's incompatible with other aspects of your body? This section addresses those issues.

No man (or woman) is an island, wrote John Donne more than 400 years ago, and it remains true today. We are individuals, but we come from families, and we carry with us remnants of those origins throughout our lives—in our bodies and in our psyches. Chapter 12 looks at how our genetic and emotional heritage affects the way we look and eat and feel.

It's not just what you eat but *how* you eat it that determines how well a diet will work for you. Do you skip meals frequently? Do you snack when you are bored? Are you a stress eater? Do you overeat at parties? Eating habits can contribute mightily to difficulties you have in maintaining the weight you desire. In chapter 13, I'll address some bad eating habits and offer strategies for modifying them.

Then, in chapter 14 we look at your lifestyle and how it may contribute to the difficulties you have in losing weight or maintaining your optimal weight. Do you eat out more than you eat in? That's a problem, because restaurants tend to load your plate with fattening foods. Do you work so many hours that any nonwork activity— eating and exercising included—is squeezed out of your life? Are you chronically sleep-deprived? These are barriers to your being able to achieve and maintain an optimal weight. We'll identify your blocks to weight loss and maintenance and discuss some ways of overcoming them.

Let's get started on designing a program to work just for you.

# CHAPTER 9
# FOOD PREFERENCES

## CARNIMORE

*"Red meat is not bad for you. Now blue-green meat, that's bad for you!"* —Tommy Smothers

If you had 5 servings or more of meat and eggs in your diary, then you are probably a Carnimore, that is, someone who enjoys eating meat. Despite its bad reputation, there is nothing wrong with making meat part of your diet and plenty of things right with doing so, but as with everything else in life, there are better and worse ways to do this.

When you think about meat as nutrition, you are really thinking about two fundamental food categories: protein and fat. Let's talk about each of them separately, and then—because we do not eat food components but food itself—we'll put it all back together with recommendations on how to eat meat in a way that is healthy.

## Protein: The Good News

Here, in a nutshell, is why protein is so important.

- Protein is the basic building block of all of our body structures and most of the messengers that make our bodies work.

- Meat provides complete proteins that contain all of the amino acids we need to manufacture more proteins that keep our bodies running.

- A diet rich in protein protects muscle mass when you are losing weight.

- Protein intake promotes bone growth. Weight loss causes bone loss, but research has shown that eating a diet that has up to 450 calories a day of protein will help decrease bone loss associated with losing weight.

- Protein makes you feel full. Many studies have been done on the so-called sating effect of foods—that is, how satisfied different foods make you feel—and when fats, carbs, and proteins are compared, proteins make you feel full quicker and longer. That's a really big plus.

So how much protein do we need? Well, 97 percent of the population would get enough protein if they ate only 0.3 gram of protein for every pound of body weight. If you look at this in terms of food, it translates into one 6-ounce steak if you weigh 150 pounds. That's per day. That's all.

You Carnimores are probably howling at this point. Remember, that's the minimum. What's the optimal level? The current thinking is that those who are limiting their calories to lose weight should eat at least 2 grams per 3 pounds of body weight, about double the minimum amount recommended.

So, are you Carnimores who eat more than the allotted protein in trouble? The Harvard Nurses' Study looked at protein intake and risk of heart disease and found that the women who took in the most protein—25 percent of their calories every day—had a lower risk of heart disease than women who ate the least amount of protein. And even those who consumed the least meat still ate considerably more than the minimum.

So, why not go on an all-protein diet?

## Protein: The Bad News

High-protein diets, which are very hot right now, want you to replace your pasta and sandwiches with just the meaty toppings and fillings. Any recent fashion magazine is likely to have a story about a model or starlet who has lost weight by eating only meat or fish. It seems to work for many—so, to quote an old burger ad, Where's the beef?

The biggest flaw is this: We doctors worry about the kidneys. Proteins are broken down to their smaller units, amino acids, and those are used throughout the body. Your body can't store protein, so if you eat more than you use, the leftovers have to be broken down and eliminated. That's done, in large part, by the kidneys, and the concern is that a diet too high in protein could strain your kidneys.

In laboratories, researchers have watched what happens to the body after a high protein load. Four hours afterward, more blood is directed to the kidneys, which suggests that they are working harder. So, does working harder definitely mean hurting? Not necessarily, at least not for healthy kidneys. But people who have even a small degree of kidney disease should not eat a high-protein diet. If you have any concerns about how well your kidneys work, you should check with your doctor before ratcheting up the amount of protein in your diet—since you already eat a fair amount of this stuff. And since protein is also broken down in the liver, those with significant liver disease do not do well on a high-protein diet either.

Since you already eat a diet high in protein, Carnimore that you are, you need to make sure you have enough water in your system to keep your kidneys working well as they get rid of waste. This is one of the major reasons everyone is always told to drink a lot of water— and it is particularly true for Carnimores. Eight glasses of water every day should do the trick.

The other issue for you meat eaters is what you *aren't* getting when you eat nothing but proteins: fiber, vitamins, and antioxidants. These are the components of foods that make it good for you. All three are necessary for good health, and these three in particular also prevent disease, including heart disease and cancer. Most protein sources are sorely lacking in these dietary components, yet no diet can be complete without them.

The final problem with a diet that depends too completely on protein has nothing to do with the protein itself and everything to do with another food component frequently linked to it: fat. You know the story here, and you know I'm not saying that all fat is evil. The fact of the matter is that saturated fats, which are the predominant fat in meats, are linked to high cholesterol and heart disease.

## Cholesterol and Heart Disease

How does a diet high in saturated fat cause high cholesterol? It's not known exactly, but here's the theory: When we eat fat and cholesterol, it goes to the liver. Then it's shipped around to the places it needs to go in our bodies by little "taxi" proteins—the most important of which are known as LDL. Something about saturated fats makes it harder for these LDL taxis to deliver the fat to the cells where it's needed. This means the LDL and its fat and cholesterol cargo spend a lot more time in the blood vessels where they're not supposed to be.

Eventually, some of the LDL taxis just dump their load right there in the vessel and not inside the cells where it belongs. It forms a layer of fat on the inside walls of the vessels. This fat layer becomes the foundation for atherosclerosis (hardening of the arteries), and that contributes to heart disease. Trans fats probably work the same way.

Unsaturated fats don't have this problem. They are easily taken up by cells. They don't cause atherosclerotic disease and may actually work to reduce the damage caused by saturated fats. How? A diet high in mono- and polyunsaturated fats gives us more of a different kind of fat taxi known as HDL cholesterol. HDL is known as the good cholesterol because it doesn't deliver fat; it retrieves fat. This tiny taxi goes out into the body and collects excess cholesterol from the arteries and cells and brings it back to the liver where it can be used as energy or shipped out for storage.

And what about omega fats? How are they good for you? When these fats are used to build cells, they make them stronger and less likely to be damaged. It's damage to artery cells that causes heart attacks, so eating a lot of omega fats can make you less likely to get heart disease. Carnimores who eat fish and grass-fed beef may end up with high levels of HDL (good) cholesterol, and that will protect them from heart disease.

## What About Eggs?

If cholesterol is the link between saturated fats and heart disease, aren't eggs, which are chock-full of cholesterol, bad for you? Way back in the twentieth century, weren't we told to avoid cholesterol-containing foods—like eggs? Yes, we were, but that connection was probably due to a simplistic understanding of how our bodies work. Cholesterol is a very important substance. Many of our hormones are made of cholesterol—testosterone and estrogen being two of the most familiar—but cortisol, adrenaline, and other very essential hormones are also made from it. Our bodies can make cholesterol, but we also get it through diet. If you eat less cholesterol, you make more of it. If you eat more, you make less. The concern comes when you eat too much cholesterol.

When researchers were first investigating the link between cholesterol and heart disease, it seemed clear that lowering cholesterol was one way to decrease risk of heart disease. And it seemed reasonable that limiting intake of dietary cholesterol would help people lower their total cholesterol. Reasonable, but not true. It's one of the wonders of our bodies (and the state of our current knowledge) that things that seem absolutely logical, given what we know, don't turn out to be right. So it was with cholesterol. As the case against saturated fats became clearer, the role of dietary cholesterol became less so. Was having a high dietary cholesterol level really linked with increased risk of heart disease independent of saturated fat? Well, as it turns out, probably not. And eating moderate amounts of eggs does not seem to increase risk of heart disease.

Of course, there's been a study looking at this. Published in 1999 in *JAMA*, this study followed the course of tens of thousands of people who ate eggs. Some ate them daily, some weekly, some monthly. It was clear that eating up to seven eggs per week, even over years, did not increase their risk of heart disease—so it probably won't increase yours either.

That's not that surprising when you know how much good stuff is in an egg. Eggs are low in saturated fats, high in monounsaturated fats, high in protein, and high in calcium, B vitamins, and vitamin A. The cholesterol is found exclusively in the yolk; the white is mostly protein. So we welcome the egg back to a healthy diet with open arms—and mouths.

# FAT CONTENT OF COMMON MEATS

| Type of Meat | Fat (g per serving) | Saturated Fat (g per serving) | Notes |
|---|---|---|---|
| Beef | 9 | 5 | Low-fat (cheaper) cuts have somewhat less, and fancy cuts (sirloin, T-bone, etc.) and organ meats have more. Hamburger, even the "lower-fat" varieties, has the most fat of all. |
| Lamb | 6 | 2 | Legs have less, chops have more. Ground lamb contains up to twice as much fat as the regular cuts. |
| Pork | 7 | 3 | Low-fat cuts (Canadian bacon and ham) contain as little as 1 gram per serving. |
| Chicken (skin removed) | 4 | 1 | If you eat the skin, add another 2 grams of fat. |
| Fish (most fish and seafood) | 1–2 | Less than 1 | |
| Fish—high fat (includes catfish, salmon, pompano, tilefish) | 5–10 | 3 | In general, wild fish contains 5 grams of fat; farm-bred fish contains twice as much fat. |

On a low-carb diet, Carnimores who like eggs may find themselves eating more than seven eggs per week. If that sounds like you, try combining one egg yolk with two egg whites to increase the protein and decrease the cholesterol.

## Eating Meat and Eggs: The Plan

So, what's a Carnimore to do?

Here's my advice: Go ahead and eat eggs, meat, or fish once or twice a day. But—there's always a but, isn't there?—give yourself a good variety of these foods. Specifically, limit your saturated fats and try to eat more fish and seafood.

How much saturated fat is allowed? The current recommendation from the National Cholesterol Education Program is that you eat less than 200 milligrams of cholesterol per day and that less than 7 percent of your calories come from saturated fats. Seven percent. So if you were eating a 1,200-calorie diet, that would allow you 10 grams of saturated fat. If you eat 1,500 calories, you can have 12 grams of saturated fat. If you eat a 1,000-calorie diet, you can have just 8 grams of saturated fat per day.

Here is a list of some foods and how much saturated fat they contain. Notice that cheese is on this list for you Carnimores because it is very high in saturated fat and is often served with meat. A tiny amount of cheese can fill your allotment for the day. You don't have to get rid of it, you just need to know and take it into consideration as you think about what you are eating.

| | |
|---|---|
| Chicken (4 oz) | 4 grams |
| Lamb | 4 grams |
| Pork | 3–4 grams |
| Beef (4 oz) | 5 grams |
| Fish (4 oz) | 3–4 grams |
| Egg (1 whole) | 2 grams |

| | |
|---|---|
| Ice cream (½ cup) | 0–4 grams (Really depends on the brand so look at the label) |
| Cheese (1 oz) | 4–8 grams |

## Tips for Carnimores, No Matter What Diet You Are On

1. Use lower-fat cuts. These are usually the cheaper cuts: chuck, loin, top or bottom round, and ribs. The fancier stuff often has a higher fat content: roasts, sirloin, tenderloin, and organ meats. And skip the ground meats—if you need it, buy a regular cut and have it ground for you.

2. Remember that, in general, beef has more saturated fat than most cuts of pork, which has more fat than most poultry, which has more saturated fat than most types of seafood.

3. When you use lower-fat cuts of meat, they can be a little dry. Don't cook them too long (a meat thermometer helps), and consider marinating in advance or adding a little pico de gallo or other low-fat sauce to the meat to boost the flavor.

4. Try new lower-fat gourmet meats and poultry. New gourmet grass-fed cuts of beef have less saturated fat and more omega-3 fatty acids than the corn-fed beef you usually get at the supermarket. Free-range chickens have less fat overall and less saturated fat. And although they tend to be expensive, they're much tastier and healthier for you.

5. When you cook the meat, make sure you do not increase the saturated fat content by adding butter. Cuts or varieties that need added fats should be cooked with olive oil.

6. Eat seafood as often as you can. Omega-3 fatty acids are linked to lower cardiac risks. When you eat seafood, choose wild fish over farm-bred fish when you can. The wild variety is much lower in fat. Plus, mercury and PCBs and all the other chemicals we worry about in fish are even lower in the wild types. Take off the skin before eating to further reduce your chance of exposure to any pollutants.

7. Portion is learned. So when you crave a steak or some other form of meat, measure your portion; 3 to 4 ounces looks small to us, because we have been trained to expect an 8-ounce or even a 12-ounce steak. Don't let your eyes talk you into a bigger piece of meat because it's what you are used to. Teach yourself a new portion size. Figure out what you want, not what advertisers tell you that you want.

## KNOW YOUR FATS

Fats can be lumped into two groups: the "bad" fats, which increase your risk of heart disease, stroke, and some cancers; and the "good" fats, which can reduce those risks.

### The Bad Fats

- Saturated fats: These are found primarily in meats and dairy products. The white stuff at the edge of your steak?—That's it.
- Trans fats: These fats are found in many margarines and shortenings and provide a smooth, creamy texture to many cookies, crackers, and pastries on the grocery store shelf. They should be on the label, but you can also find them in the ingredients list as "partially hydrogenated fatty acids."

### The Good Fats

- Monounsaturated fats: These are most abundant in olive oil and canola oil. They are also found in all nuts and in some high-fat foods from the fruits and vegetables group, such as avocado. Small amounts are also found in lean meats and fish.
- Polyunsaturated fats: These are found in most vegetable oils—corn oil, peanut oil, sunflower seed oil—and in nuts.
- Omega fats: These are most abundant in fish and seafood. They are also found in beef that is grass-fed (as opposed to the corn-fed beef we usually see).

**For carbohydrate counters:** Eggs contain virtually no carbohydrate and so are a perfect food for this diet. They do, however, contain some saturated fats and lots of cholesterol. Where possible, consider using one yolk with two whites when you need to cook with eggs. The yolk contains all the cholesterol and most of the calories; the white is mostly protein.

**For calorie counters:** Mostly because of the fat, meat tends to have a high calorie count. This is where portion control becomes essential. Try buying cuts of meat that are naturally small. For instance, use chicken or turkey cutlets rather than chicken breasts. Lamb chops, while relatively high in fat, are small, and one or two tiny ones may fill your need for meat. Beef comes in thin cutlets, too. They have a variety of names; where I live they are called minute steaks. Utilizing these tricks, you won't have to use as much willpower to maintain your portion control.

**For fat counters:** If eating red meat only once or twice a week seems like a hardship, try working in small amounts of meat more often. A serving is usually 3 to 4 ounces. Try dividing those small portions into even smaller portions and eating meat more frequently. You can make a great-tasting roast beef sandwich loaded with tomatoes, sprouts, lettuce, onions, horseradish, and whatever else you like, using only 1 ounce of meat. Or try adding a small amount of meat to a vegetable stir-fry to reduce the amount of meat in your diet without making you feel deprived.

Use recipes that incorporate meat as an ingredient in a dish rather than featuring meat as the centerpiece of your meal. Where possible, reduce by one-half the amount of meat that's called for in regular recipes.

# MILK MAVIN

*"Things are seldom what they seem, skim milk masquerades as cream."* —Sir William Schwenk Gilbert, *H.M.S. Pinafore*

## Dairy Products: The Good News

If you ate more than 6 servings of dairy products in your diet diary, you are likely a Milk Mavin. The world of nutrition has had mixed feelings about milk over the past couple of decades, and as a result milk, which used to be considered the very epitome of a health food, is now viewed with some suspicion. In the 1950s and before, the model was the four food groups, so milk and dairy products were touted as foods that should be eaten every day.

Then in the 1970s and 1980s, researchers started looking into sources of cholesterol and saturated fat in the diet, and it was clear that for many Americans butter, cheeses, and whole milk were as important a source of these dietary demons as red meat. So, Americans were advised to eschew butter and replace it with margarine. The advice with respect to milk was to avoid it as much as possible, and if you couldn't avoid it, then to make sure that the milk that you drank was skim—a grayish, watery liquid, difficult to enjoy after the rich whiteness of whole milk.

If you look at the previous USDA food pyramid, published in 1992, you'll find dairy products near the skinny top of the pyramid along with other foods that may be in your diet in small amounts. That status is starting to change again and in the newest version of the food pyramid milk is listed as one of five categories of must-have foods.

So, what good comes from dairy products? A lot. First and foremost, for those of us who want to live to a ripe old age, dairy products are an important source of dietary calcium, and calcium is important for the protection of our bones. Since weight loss in and of itself causes bone loss, it's especially important that you do what you can to build up bone mineral density. Research shows that drinking milk is a good way to do that.

Eating dairy products has other health benefits as well. For example, diets rich in dairy products lower blood pressure and reduce risk of stroke. Diets high in dairy products have also been linked with lower rates of colon cancer. Some very interesting data suggest that calcium supplements decrease the salt cravings that torment so many women before their periods. Most compelling is research that suggests that people who eat a high level of dairy products are less likely to be overweight than those with lower intakes. This may be related to an associated decrease in consumption of soft drinks, one of the most common sources of sugar in our diet. But there is evidence that milk and other dairy products contain something that promotes less weight gain—although what, exactly, is not clear.

## Dairy Products: The Bad News

As with all things nutritional, there is also a downside—milk products can contain high levels of saturated fats. Check the label to find out if the milk you drink contains saturated fat. And many people are lactose intolerant. There are degrees of lactose intolerance, and if you're lucky, then Lactaid might work for you. Lactase pills can cover you if you really want a pizza with cheese or an occasional ice cream sandwich.

Those with significant lactose intolerance, who get the symptoms when they even *think* about milk, should remember that some milk products, like yogurt, can be eaten without developing symptoms, because they bring their own bacteria. Also, remember that only cow's milk causes the problem. Milks and cheeses from other animals don't. Soy products, while they don't have the same type of benefits as dairy products, have their own pluses. If soy milk and soy ice cream taste good to you, dig in.

## Tips for Milk Mavins, No Matter What Diet You Are On

1. If you are going to drink milk and can't bear the taste of the grayish fluid known as skim (or fat-free) milk, buy 1% milk. It has about 2 grams of fat per cup (so about 20 percent of its calories come from fat) and only 10 calories more than the fat-free version. It also tastes and looks about a million times better. If you use milk in your coffee, you'll also end up using less of it if you use 1% milk instead of skim.

2. When you are cooking with cheese, you can often substitute reduced-fat cheeses without affecting the flavor of the dish.

3. Limit your intake of high-fat cheeses, but when you do eat them, eat a moderate amount and try to reduce the amount of fat in the other parts of your diet that day.

4. Use butter just for flavoring, and when you use it, do it sparingly. You might try butter spray instead of the usual stick stuff. It's easier to use less.

5. Use low-fat sour cream instead of regular; the taste is pretty good.

6. Substitute low-fat or fat-free frozen yogurt for the ice cream you crave.

**For carbohydrate counters:** Don't use fat-free dairy products. In general, fat is replaced with carbohydrates in reduced-fat foods, and dairy products are no exception. On the other hand, lower-fat versions of many of these foods often have an acceptable amount of carbohydrate in them. Check out the label.

**For calorie counters:** If you like your yogurt flavored, buy low-fat or light yogurt in the smallest containers. These usually contain around 6 ounces of yogurt and give you enough to enjoy while limiting your portion.

**For fat counters:** The fat in milk and dairy products is mostly saturated and the stuff you want to limit the most. So always use the low-fat or fat-free version of your favorite dairy product. If they seem thin or watery to you, try stepping down the fat content one step at a time. For example, if you drink whole milk, switch to 2%, which looks and tastes like whole. Then move to 1% milk. Finally, try fat-free. If the pale, gray fluid is a turnoff, try fat-free milk fortified with "nonfat milk solids," which has a better look and a creaminess that makes it taste and feel like it has fat in it.

## CALORIE, FAT, AND CARB CONTENT OF ORDINARY CHEESES

| Cheese | Calories | Fat (g) | Carbohydrate (g) |
|---|---|---|---|
| Cottage cheese, low-fat, ½ cup | 90 | 1–5 | 4 |
| Feta cheese, 1 oz | 75 | 6 | 1 |
| Mozzarella, whole milk, 1 oz | 80 | 6 | 1 |
| Mozzarella, reduced-fat, 1 oz | 72 | 3 | 1 |
| Ricotta, reduced-fat, ¼ cup | 64 | 3 grams per oz | 2 grams per oz |
| String cheese, 1 oz | 80 | 1 | 5 |

# VEGECARIAN

*"Don't be afraid to go out on a limb—that's where the fruit is."*
—Father Andrew SDC

If you recorded eating more than 8 fruit and vegetable servings in your food diary, then you may very well be what I call a VegeCarian, and that's wonderful. Fruits and vegetables are good for you and should be at the heart of just about any diet.

## Fruits and Vegetables: The Good News

Your mother has been harping on the benefits of fruits and veggies since you were a kid, so you may not think it's possible for me to come up with any new information on this front. Let me give it a shot.

**Fruits and vegetables are a low-calorie, high-nutrient-value food.** A diet high in fruits and vegetables will promote weight loss, because these foods contain plenty of water and not so many calories. This is particularly important for those of you who need a lot of food to feel full.

Let me introduce you to the idea of energy density. Basically, that's how many calories a food contains per unit of volume. As it turns out, for many of us, how much food we eat is an important aspect of feeling full. Eating foods with a low energy density allows us to eat satisfying portions of food and still take in fewer calories. Barbara Rolls, Ph.D., a researcher at Pennsylvania State University, made an important observation a few years ago, an observation that may seem obvious but had never been demonstrated before: Most of us eat about the same volume of food each day. What makes up that volume changes from day to day, but the amount stays pretty stable. What this means is that if you eat the same volume but consume fewer calories, you will feel full but will lose weight.

So, what kinds of foods have lower energy density? Generally, these are foods with a high water content, so fruits and vegetables are front and center. Let me give you an example of how this works: You eat a bowl of pasta for dinner. A 2-ounce serving of pasta—that's just over 200 calories—and a light sprinkle of olive oil and Parmesan cheese—that's another 200 calories—and there you have a small serving of pasta. Two ounces of cooked pasta, depending on which type you cook, is about ¼ cup. So your 400-calorie meal is tiny. But if you decided instead to add some fresh tomatoes to the pasta, you could sauté the tomato in the olive oil you were going to add to your pasta anyway, then maybe you'd add some onions, squash, and mushrooms. You could double the amount of food you eat, triple it even, and add fewer than 50 calories. But, chances are, you'd feel a lot fuller after the second dish than the first dish. (Of course, that's a fake argument because you'd probably eat a larger serving of that first one anyway!) Adding vegetables contributes to your sense of satiety without contributing to calories. Now, that's a bargain.

**Fruits and veggies are high in fiber, and fiber promotes weight loss.** As you know, fruits and vegetables have lots of fiber. At its most basic level, fiber is the stuff in fruits and vegetables that isn't starch and that's hard to digest. You can't absorb fiber, so it is the calorie-free portion of food. There are two kinds of fiber, and they are both good for you, albeit in different ways. Soluble fiber turns to jelly in your stomach. As such, it promotes a sense of fullness, and it slows the absorption of sugar and other nutrients so that your glucose level has less of a tendency to get out of hand. Soluble fiber is found in foods like oats. Diets high in soluble fiber have been found to decrease risk of heart disease.

Insoluble fiber passes through your digestive system virtually untouched. However, in transit it performs a vital job: It promotes stool bulk and causes water to be absorbed by the lower intestines, moving food through and preventing constipation. This is important to everyone, but especially those on a carbohydrate-counting diet, since constipation is a frequent side effect. High-fiber diets reduce the risk of some cancers and help prevent diverticular disease.

Finally, fruits, vegetables, and other high-fiber foods may help you lose weight by increasing your body's production of a hormone called Peptide YY. When obese and thin people are given injections of this protein (as explained in a recent study published in *The New*

*England Journal of Medicine*), they ate much less food over the next 24 hours. Researchers believe that a high-fiber diet, which increases your Peptide YY level, will also make you feel less hungry.

**Fruits and vegetables promote weight loss.** Because fruits and vegetables have a lower energy density than most other foods, eating these foods rather than something else will promote weight loss. And most fruits and vegetables are very low glycemic–load foods, so they not only provide bulk with fewer calories but they are easy on your insulin level as well, which may help you lose weight, too.

There are, of course, exceptions to this rule. Potatoes have a high glycemic load (GL). One serving of a baked potato has a GL of 26, much higher than the GL of peas (3), carrots (2), or cherries (3). That puts potatoes in the same category as some cakes, cookies, or fruit roll-ups. Does this mean you can't have potatoes? No, but it means that you should limit your potato intake, and when you do eat them, add a low-fat protein to slow down the glycemic load. Low-fat or fat-free sour cream does a nice job. Other low-fat cheeses work as well. Or add some salsa with or without a touch of olive oil. And, of course, lower your intake of French fries. Most fast-food varieties are fried in oils high in trans fats, so they are a double nutritional debit.

**Beta-carotene and other antioxidants prevent disease.** You know these are good for you, but do you know why? The way your body is damaged and ages is through oxidation, a perfectly natural process. (On the other hand, so is dying. So if we can fight it, we should.) Dietary antioxidants in the form of fruits and vegetables look like one way to do just that. In one study, folks who ate at least 5 servings of these foods a day lived longer (and were thinner) than those who ate less. But you can't take the healthy ingredients and put them in a pill and get the same benefit. Studies have shown that antioxidant supplements will not provide the same protection as their fruit and vegetable sources.

**Vitamins and minerals are essential for health.** Carbohydrates, proteins, and fats are the basic categories of foods that we eat; they are called macronutrients, because they are the energy and building blocks of our bodies. In many foods there are other important components that we call micronutrients. We need only tiny amounts of these components, but they are essential for many of the biological processes that go on in our bodies. We need all of these micronutrients, and when we don't get them, we get sick. Many of these come from the fruits and veggies you eat.

Some of the ways fruits and vegetables are treated reduces their nutritional value. Canned foods have lower nutritional value than frozen foods. Frozen foods have lower value than fresh foods. Some ways of cooking are better than others. For example, boiling foods can leach some of the nutrients into the water, which is discarded. Steaming or sautéing avoids this problem. On the other hand, eating these foods any way you can get them is better than not having them, so don't let availability or cooking preference interfere with your eating them.

**A special word about nuts:** Nuts are not usually considered in a chapter about fruits and vegetables, but I would argue that they ought to be. Nuts are a nutrient-dense food that I think should be made part of a healthy diet. Yes, they are high in calories, they are also high in fiber, high in high-quality protein, and high in polyunsaturated fats.

Studies have shown that a diet high in nuts can improve lipids and reduce the risk of heart disease and diabetes. And although nuts have lots of calories and usually lots of salt, they are also high in their ability to sate appetite. (So, eat nuts, but avoid bingeing on them.)

## How Much Is Enough?

The new food pyramid recommends that we eat 4–6 cups of fruits and vegetables every day—depending on level on physical activity. I would go further than that. If you like these foods, this group is the one type of food that I would say "more is better." These low-glycemic-index fruits and vegetables can and should be eaten freely. So 4–6 cups per day is a good goal, but if you want more, eat more, unless you're on the 30-gram Counting Carbohydrates Diet. Folks who are limiting their carbs to 30 grams or less a day will get only a few servings of vegetables and fruits per day. But, remember, that stage of the diet is only for a couple of months. Any longer than that and it becomes much less effective. So the ban on fruit and veggie gorging is brief.

## Is There Any Bad News About Fruits and Vegetables?

No. Not from my perspective. Some people are concerned about increasing their exposure to the pesticides used in growing these foods. I have actually found very little U.S.-published data on this from the past 10 years. Studies done more than 10 years ago showed no residue on most foods, and those with some residues were well within USDA/FDA standards. Within the past 10 years, there has also been a great deal of literature from outside the United States. These studies have also shown either no or small residues on foods, all within USDA/FDA standards.

I think the strongest argument for the healthiness of fruits and vegetables lies in the studies showing that folks who eat more fruits and veggies are healthier (not to mention thinner) than those who eat fewer. So, if you like these foods, eat up!

## Tips for VegeCarians, No Matter What Diet You Are On

1. Aim for at least 5 servings of vegetables and 4 servings of fruit per day.

2. Buy fresh vegetables whenever you can. Only use the canned or frozen stuff when what you want isn't available fresh.

3. When choosing a fruit or vegetable for a snack, make sure you pair it up with a protein to make the snack last. Far too often, people will snack on an apple or carrots several hours before they plan to eat a meal and then find they are hungry an hour or two later. Eating a protein with your carb will give the snack the staying power you need to get you to your next meal without hunger. On the next page I have listed some low-fat snacks that add up to 200 calories or less.

**For carbohydrate counters:** Getting your fill of vegetables and fruits is going to be tough in the early phase of your Counting Carbs Diet, when both serving size and variety are extremely limited. It's easy to eat just a simple salad with your favorite dressing every day. But if you do that, you'll be so bored that it will be hard for you to eat even the limited amount you're allowed.

Try different salad dressings to liven up your salad. Most are low in carbohydrates. And, try different salads as well. Too often we put just about everything we have in the kitchen into the salad. Try focusing on only one or two flavors in your salad. It increases the variety in your diet. Try a tomato and cucumber salad. How about a hearts of palm salad? Endive can make a fast interesting salad. In making these more flavor-focused salads, you can give yourself a greater spectrum of tastes and it's also a lot less work.

When you're going to cook your veggies, don't just steam them. Try sautéing vegetables with a tiny bit of olive oil. Add garlic, chile peppers, and stock or white wine. Casseroles that use eggs and cheese with veggies make a nice change as well. Recipes that show you how to cook the low-carb way can be found at the end of chapter 6.

**For calorie counters:** Look for new and interesting fruits and vegetables to add to your repertoire. One of the biggest problems with the way many of us eat veggies is boredom. Be adventurous—try new foods and new recipes often. You can start with the recipes at the end of chapter 7.

## LOW-FAT SNACK COMBINATIONS

| Snack | Calories | Fat (g) | Carbohydrate (g) |
|---|---|---|---|
| Cantaloupe with 8 oz fat-free, plain yogurt | 146 | 0.2 | 25 |
| Cucumber (1), sliced, and 2 tbsp hummus | 97 | 3.4 | 11 |
| Jell-O, sugar-free, ½ cup | 8 | 0 | 0 |
| Peach (1), sliced, with ½ cup 1% cottage cheese | 158 | 1.1 | 21 |
| Popcorn, light butter-flavored, 3 cups | 60 | 2 | 12 |
| Potato chips, baked, 1 oz | 110 | 5 | 23 |
| Seven-grain bread, 1 slice, with 2 tsp apple butter | 105 | 21 | 1.2 |
| Tomato (1), large, with 1 oz string cheese | 118 | 5.4 | 7 |

**For fat counters:** Rather than slathering your veggies with butter, try other sauces and flavors to spice up the same old steamed veggies: Lemon juice is an old favorite; curry powder (especially homemade) can really add punch; a vinaigrette can also work well; fat-free pestos will liven up an otherwise plain dish. For more ideas, see the recipes at the end of chapter 8.

## STARCH STEALER

*"What I say is that, if a man really likes potatoes, he must be a pretty decent sort of fellow."* —A. A. Milne

*"Everything you see I owe to spaghetti."*—Sophia Loren

If you ate 8 or more servings of these foods, then chances are good that you are a Starch Stealer. Welcome to the club. It's a very big club indeed. Most of the people in the world get most of their calories from these types of foods. Even in this country, where we are berated for eating so much fat, we continue to eat a diet that's dominated by starchy carbohydrates.

These starchy carbs are the newest nutritional battleground. There are entire sections of diet books dedicated to "carbohydrate addicts" and their "carbohydrate cravings." And I know these cravings are real: I have patients who tell me they dream about bread and potatoes and rice when they are on a diet that forbids these foods. Despite the clamorous confusion and our limited (though rapidly growing) knowledge, let's try to make sense of it.

## Starches: The Good News

When doctors and nutritionists advocate a way of eating that they believe will promote health and weight loss for most people, they usually recommend a low-fat, high-carbohydrate diet. What that means is that we should get fewer of our calories from fats and meats and more of our calories from pasta, rice, bread, and potatoes as well as fruits and vegetables. If you look at the old USDA food pyramid on page 120, you will see that at the bottom of the graphic, the food group we should eat the most of is breads and other starches. That hasn't changed—we're still exhorted to eat 6–10 ounces of grains per day. Those recommendations were based on strong epidemiological evidence that this way of eating is associated with a lower risk of obesity and heart disease.

Many of these foods are low in calories and high in nutrition. They are also high in bulk. They take up room in your stomach so you can fill up without consuming too many calories, and that's important.

Starches and other carbohydrates are also easily converted to glucose, the preferred body fuel. When you eat these foods, you are providing the energy your brain and body need in the form they like the best. And that's good.

Finally, research has shown that many people prefer eating high-carb foods—especially sweets—when they are stressed. In a study done in London, researchers recruited sixty-eight healthy men and women to participate in an investigation of "the effects of hunger on physiology, performance, and mood." Half were told that they would be expected to give a 4-minute speech after lunch and were given 10 minutes to prepare a talk on an assigned topic. The other half was instructed to listen to a tape on which a man read poetry by Dylan Thomas.

After 10 minutes at each activity, the group was reunited and served lunch. Blood pressure, heart rate, and mood were assessed for each person before and after the 10-minute activity. It's important to say that not everyone in the speech group felt stressed by the task. Stress isn't just what happens, but how we respond to it.

At lunch, there were a variety of foods available from which each participant was free to choose. The amount each person ate during the first 15 minutes of the meal was carefully measured. Those who were stressed by their speech-preparation task ate a higher proportion of sweets and fats and consumed more calories than those who didn't feel stressed. Why did the stress generated by the anxiety about giving a speech cause the subjects to choose starchy (and fat-laden) foods?

Research suggests that for some people, eating carbohydrates can actually stabilize their moods by changing the chemicals in their brains. For these people, starchy carbs are an instant antidote for stress. They should be on a low-fat, high-carb diet so they can incorporate their needed carbohydrates into their daily meals and snacks.

## Starches: The Bad News

One of the problems with starches is that they are very easy to overeat. They are often warm and somewhat bland in taste, and they just feel good going down. Because of this, I recommend that you try serving yourself modest portions of these yummy foods initially. If you are still hungry, you can go back for more. Basically, I want you to *un*-supersize it and see what it really takes to make you feel full. For instance, a serving of pasta is 2 ounces. A serving of cooked rice is ½ cup, and a serving of potatoes is one medium-size potato or ½ cup.

Finally, when you are preparing your starchy meal or snack, keep energy density in mind. You can eat ½ cup of pasta with a little red sauce, and that might make you feel full, or you could spice it up with some very low density foods—mushrooms, green peppers, and squash steamed or sautéed in a tiny amount of olive oil. That combination will increase the amount of food you eat without increasing the number of calories much. It allows you to have your starch and eat it, too. And (need I even say this?) when you are eating a naturally low-density starch, don't make it denser by deep-fat frying it or covering it with fat; make it *less* dense by adding fiber or vegetables to it so that a little carbohydrate can really take you a long way.

## Tips for Starch Stealers, No Matter What Diet You Are On

1. Choose low-glycemic-load starches over those with a high glycemic load. For a list of foods and their glycemic loads, see page 124.

2. When your starch craving comes from stress, think about other ways to manage your stress. Trying to deal with the cause of stress may be the best way to get rid of your craving. Take a walk and think about why you really need that donut or cookie. That often gets rid of the craving as well as the stress.

3. When you have a starch as part of a meal, serve yourself a modest portion and go back for seconds if you are still hungry.

## WHY STRESS MAKES YOU CRAVE CARBS

Researchers at MIT in the 1970s found that carbohydrate consumption by rats promoted the production of serotonin in their brains. This is how it works: Carbs increase insulin; insulin makes cells take up glucose and most amino acids (the most basic component of proteins). One amino acid that is not taken up by cells when insulin is around is tryptophan. Instead, tryptophan is taken up in the brain. This uptake is normally blocked by the presence of other amino acids, so having low levels of them in the blood makes it possible for tryptophan to better enter the brain, where it is converted to serotonin, an important mood stabilizer. This process initially described in rats has since been witnessed in people, too.

Researchers set up a live-in facility at MIT and invited overweight men and women to stay there while they studied them. What they ate was carefully monitored in their own special cafeteria, and they were able to snack as they wanted using specially designed vending machines. They were given a "credit" card that allowed them to choose whatever they desired from the machines: fruit, candy, cookies, chips, yogurt—you name it.

After a couple of weeks, the researchers looked at what the live-in subjects had eaten, and an interesting pattern emerged. Many of them would eat normally at mealtimes, but then take in almost as many calories with snacks from the vending machines. Most of these snacks were high-carbohydrate foods. Moreover, these people did not eat snacks all day long, but tended to eat the same kind of foods at the same time each day. Later interviews with the subjects showed that the stimulus for the snack was a mood change and that eating the snack reversed the mood. The researchers concluded that these folks were using the carbohydrates as a drug to treat their bad feelings.

**For carbohydrate counters:** I can only recommend starches as a very occasional treat. One of the ways this diet works is by limiting the foods you can eat and in that way limiting the calories you take in. On the other hand, if you crave an occasional starch, who am I to criticize? Just consider them the once-in-a-while treats, rather than daily fare. However, avoid the "low-carb" versions of these foods. If you are going to cheat, do it with foods that are really worth it and savor the experience so it lasts. That way, you won't feel like cheating again for quite a while.

**For calorie counters:** With this type of food, portion control is tough. One trick that works for some of my patients is to eat the starch at the end of the meal, not at the beginning. Start with the protein-containing food and the vegetable, and then finish with the starch. It's much easier not to overeat when you are almost full.

**For fat counters:** Many starches come attached to fats, often saturated fats. This is particularly true of sweet starches and baked goods like cookies, muffins, pastries, biscuits, or bagels. The fat can give these foods a low glycemic load but still add on the calories. And calories *always* count. Try to find substitutes for your favorite high-fat starches that will limit your calorie intake. You can try buying a smaller one of whatever it is, or try new and lower-calorie versions and see if that helps.

## SWEETS EATER

*"Chocolate is a perfect food, as wholesome as it is delicious, a beneficent restorer of exhausted power. It is the best friend of those engaged in literary pursuits."*
—Baron Justus von Liebig

*"All I really need is love, but a little chocolate now and then doesn't hurt!"* —Lucy Van Pelt (in *Peanuts*, by Charles M. Schulz)

If you recorded eating 6 or more servings of sweets in your food diary, then chances are you are a Sweets Eater. Actually, we all start off in life as Sweets Eaters; research has shown that infants instinctively prefer sweet tastes above all other tastes, and breast milk is perfectly designed to meet that demand. As a child grows, this preference decreases, but how much is variable.

While many people who struggle with their weight regret their love of sweets, I think that like anything you really love, our job is to figure out how to integrate it into a way of eating that works for you and your own taste preferences.

## Sweets: The Good News

The love of sweets is certainly built in at a very basic level. Anything that is this innate can't be all bad. In fact, a study published a few years ago suggested that moderate candy consumption, like moderate wine consumption, can prolong your life. Folks who eat one to three pieces of candy a month—I did say moderate candy consumption—can add an average of one year to their lives.

Why do we love sweets? There is good evidence that consumption of these foods can stimulate the opiate receptors, one of the primary pleasure sites we have in our brains. Researchers studying mice noted that eating sweets affected the same part of the rodents' brains that was affected by narcotics. Similar studies in humans have produced similar results.

Thus, there may be a physiologic foundation to the sense some people have that they are "addicted" to sweets. In another series of studies, mice and rats were exposed to high levels of sweet foods. When they were cut off from their supply, their little paws trembled, and they were nervous and jumpy. Basically, the researchers reported, they were going through the rodent version of withdrawal. This doesn't mean that chocolate is the same as heroin. But I think it shows that our love for sweets is part of the way we are programmed at the genetic level and not some aberration.

If a love of sweets is hardwired into the brain, willpower alone will not be enough to make you resist these cravings. You have to outsmart them.

## Sweets: The Bad News

When we look at whole populations, it becomes clear that a higher consumption of sweets is associated with higher weight. So, while fats might not make you fat, too many sweets probably will. When you separate fat consumption from sugar consumption, it's clear that a high-sweets diet is more likely to contribute to weight gain than a high-fat diet (though that's not always easy to do, since so many high-carbohydrate foods are also high-fat foods). Why is this, since sweets don't have any more calories than other foods? (In fact, sweets have only 4 calories per gram compared to fat, which has 9 calories a gram, or alcohol, which has 7 calories per gram.)

There are probably two answers. First, I think it's clear that our bodies process sugary treats differently than other foods. No other food triggers our opiate receptors. Perhaps because of this, people who love sweets tend to overeat them in a way in which they might not be tempted to overeat other foods.

In addition, there is some evidence that suggests that leptin, the hormone that is produced by fat cells to protect your fat stores, affects how things taste. High leptin levels, which are found during times of weight maintenance, are associated with a decreased preference for sweets—at least in mice. When that leptin level drops (the way it does when we humans are losing weight) the mice show a much stronger preference for sweet foods. If these findings are reproduced in humans, it will be just one more way that we are hardwired to love sweets and to use these foods to protect our precious fat stores.

From my perspective, a high-candy diet has another problem. A diet that's high in sweets is often low in fruits and vegetables. Whatever your perfect diet may be, in the long run, a diet that's high in fruits and vegetables is clearly the healthiest. Fruits and vegetables provide essential disease-fighting and cancer-preventing nutrients, they provide fiber, and they should be in everyone's diet. Unfortunately, Sweets Eaters tend to avoid fruits and vegetables.

Nevertheless I am convinced that there is a way to incorporate sweets into your diet that allows you to eat a good diet and control your weight.

## Sweets: The Plan

How you want to deal with your sweet cravings depends on how you crave them. Some people must have them every day; others want them only at times of stress; up to half of women who crave sweets do so on the days before their periods. I notice that I crave sweets only after I have had them. That is, if I eat a piece of candy, I want one the next day. If I don't eat candy for a couple of days, I won't crave it. Probably many other patterns exist, too.

There is evidence that sweets can be incorporated into a healthy diet without wreaking havoc on weight control. In Montreal, researchers took a group of people with diabetes—the very folks who are usually taught to avoid sugary sweets at all costs—and randomly divided them into two groups. One group got the usual nutritional advice; the folks in the other group were taught to allow 10 percent of their daily calories to come from sugary treats. After 6 months, the sweets eaters ate fewer calories and gained less weight than the group who got the usual teaching.

So it can be done. But you have to learn to plan around your sweets eating the same way you plan around all your other dietary goals. If you don't, and just hope for the best, then when you do succumb to your cravings (which is almost inevitable), you will be adding sweet treats on top of your full diet, and that inevitably causes weight gain.

I find that most of my patients do best when they include sweet foods into most of their meals. At breakfast, you might try peanut butter on your toast. Eat fruits at snack times and plan on having a dessert after lunch or dinner. In all my meal plans, I have included several sweets a day. The exception is the 30-gram Counting Carbohydrates Diet, where the carbohydrate limit is too low to include more than a single sweet on most days.

Try to have the sweet when you are at home, where you have arranged choices that you can feel good about. Try not to eat desserts when you eat out. Restaurant servings of sweets, like all their servings of foods, are much too large. For most people, providing sweets as part of a scheduled meal or snack reduces cravings at other times.

However, those extracurricular cravings will still come to most Sweets Eaters. When do you have most of your cravings? Most Sweets Eaters have cravings in the afternoon or evening. Researchers at MIT have also shown that many Sweets Eaters and other carb cravers tend to get their cravings at the same, predictable times each day.

This is where your food diary will come in very handy. Find out when you are most likely to crave sweets and then figure out how to satisfy your urge in a way that allows you to feel good about yourself and your weight.

When you get a craving for sweets, take a minute to think about where it's coming from. Are you stressed? Depressed? Lonely? Angry? These are common reasons I hear from my patients. See if you can take a walk, a bike ride, an exercise class. If you still have the craving after the exercise, by all means eat a treat—at least you will have burned some extra calories.

One of the patients I've told you about, Diane, came to my office not long ago, glowing with triumph. She had been tormented by cravings for sweets late at night, right before bed. She tried fruit, gum, even sugar-free candy. Nothing worked except chocolate. Still, she didn't like eating the chocolate right before bed. I had encouraged her to try exercise, and that hadn't worked either. She recognized that the craving came from a bad feeling she was having, but she couldn't figure out what she really wanted. Finally, it occurred to her that maybe she was lonely. The kids were in bed, the news on TV was all bad, she was tired, but this feeling, this longing for company kept her from going to bed. So instead of eating chocolate, she started calling her sister, also her best friend, when she felt this hunger at night. It worked, and she hadn't eaten a snack at night in more than 3 weeks. She felt empowered. She felt good.

When you get the craving for sweets, choose a sweet you can eat and still face yourself in the mirror later. Of course, that means not overeating. So, no matter which diet you are on, choose a sweet that's low in calories. If you are on a fat-counting diet, choose one that is also low in fats. If you are on a carbohydrate-counting diet, you're going to have a hard time getting any variety into your sweet treats, because most sweets are carbohydrates. Still, it can be done, and I have some tips below just for you.

You might think that a taste of what you crave is not going to be enough. You will be surprised. Sweets cravings, like many food cravings, are mediated through your mouth and its taste equipment. Your mouth has no ability to quantify how much you are eating. It only knows whether you are eating or not, so when you choose to give yourself the treat of your dreams, you can probably get away with really satisfying that craving with a much smaller serving than you are used to.

My sister Shelley loves the McDonald's treat McFlurries. There have been times in her life when she had to have one every day. But she discovered that she could order a small one and have it be just as satisfying as a large. And, more recently, there are even days when she can take a few sips and then throw the rest out, because she's satisfied.

Sweets may be the hardest food to incorporate into a rational diet, but if you are a Sweets Eater, it's important to take on that challenge. After all, it's unlikely that your preference will change, so you have to figure out a way to live with it if you want to manage your weight. The world we live in makes just saying no an unrealistic plan.

I've included a list of a few of the millions of sweet treats you might consider. Here are the qualities I look for in a treat.

- The treat should be low in calories.

- It can be purchased in small snack-size amounts.

- It comes in a form that allows you to easily understand and consume only the amount you want—for example, calorie counts that allow the snack to be divided into easily understood quantities, for example, the whole bar or this many pieces.

- It's something that you like, but not something you need to binge on; if you know you can't eat chocolate in moderation, don't buy chocolate.

## Tips for Sweets Eaters, No Matter What Diet You Are On

1. Clear the house of everything you don't want to eat. Don't just keep stuff stashed away. Get it out.

2. Always have something sweet at hand that you will feel good about eating. You can try having fruit around; very sweet fruits like grapes and melon can work for some people, at least part of the time. Frozen fruit bars might work. Low-calorie ice cream bars sometimes do the trick.

3. Have a variety of healthy sweet treats around the house and only one type of sweet that you could crave but wouldn't want to eat too much of. That will improve your odds of satisfying your craving with a food that you won't be sorry you ate.

4. Only have as much of the restricted sweet in the house as you would want to eat at any given moment. Buy serving sizes and, if necessary, buy them one at a time. Then replace your stock when you are not having cravings, so that you will be prepared next time they come.

## LOW-CALORIE SWEETS

| Sweet Treat | Calories | Fat (g) | Carbohydrate (g) |
| --- | --- | --- | --- |
| Chewing gum (most brands), 1 piece | 10 | 0 | 2 |
| D-Zerta sugar-free gelatin, ½ cup, with 3 tbsp Cool Whip | 50 | 0 | 0 |
| Frozen yogurt, light, ½ cup | 120 | 2 | 20 |
| FrozFruit popsicle | 60 | 0 | 16 |
| FrozFruit popsicle, light | 25 | 0 | 6 |
| Hershey's kisses, 6 pieces | 150 | 9 | 16 |
| Ice cream, light, ½ cup | 120 | 3 | 15 |
| Ice cream, sugar-free, ½ cup | 90 | 3 | 12 |
| Ice cream sandwich, light | 100 | 2 | 18 |
| Ice milk, ½ cup | 120 | 4 | 18 |
| Jelly beans, 10 pieces | 100 | 0 | 26 |
| Life Savers, 1 piece | 8 | 0 | 2 |
| Reese's Pieces, 10 pieces | 40 | 2 | 5 |
| Snack bar (many varieties), 1.3 oz | 140 | 5 | 20 |
| Strawberries, 1 cup, with 3 tbsp Cool Whip | 90 | 1 | 13 |
| Weight Watchers candy bar | 130 | 8 | 14 |

5. Have a plan for what to do when the wholesome sweets at hand don't do it for you. The nature of that plan will depend on you and your cravings. One of my patients, Janet, has a real sweet tooth and loves ice cream. When she craves ice cream and nothing else will do, she makes herself walk to get it. She lives in a large city, and there is a local store nearby. She figures the walk (and the hassle) into her craving calculations.

6. If you feel that you can never learn to eat sweets in moderation and decide that the only way you can deal with your "addiction" is to ban sweets forever, have a plan for what to do if you "fall off the wagon." Having no plan means leaving your diet in the hands of chance and whim. My whole shtick is that you do better in managing what you eat if you have a plan and choose what to eat, no matter how hard that is. You need to take charge of your diet, and that means staying in charge even when you can't control all your cravings all the time.

7. Finally, anticipate how you will feel after you've eaten something you hadn't planned on. Too often the response is "I'll start again tomorrow," and that can trigger a binge. Be proactive in the face of what might feel like a failure. When you are late paying a bill, you don't say, "Oh well, I'll pay that bill next month." Same with unintended splurges. Try to get back on track, that day, that hour, that very minute—and go from there.

**For carbohydrate counters:** If you love sweets, then a carbohydrate-counting diet is going to be pretty darn tough. These foods need to be eaten in moderation, especially when you are in the early phase of the diet and want to stay "in the pink." Have only a small amount of sweet foods at hand. Make sure these foods are the ones you can eat without regret.

Here are some foods you can eat in moderation, even in the early phase.

- Strawberries, blueberries, and raspberries
- Sugarless candy or gum (These snacks have a built-in overeating prevention mechanism: They can give you powerful and very regrettable gas when eaten in excess.)
- Sugarless gelatin
- A small scoop of Cool Whip or even a dab of real whipped cream to brighten up the gelatin or fruits

Remember, although sugarless items don't have carbohydrates, they do contain calories. Moderation in all things is key.

**For calorie counters:** Portion control is key in eating sweets, so give yourself an edge.

- Only have as much in the house as you would want to eat at any given moment.

- Have a variety of healthy sweet treats around and only one type of sweet that you could crave but wouldn't want to eat often. The greater the variety of sweets around you, the greater the quantity of sweets you tend to eat. Use that understanding to try to ease your craving with a variety of wholesome, low-calorie treats.

**For fat counters:** Avoid chocolate. It is loaded with fats and, in general, the higher the quality of chocolate, the greater the amount of fat, most of it saturated. If you absolutely need chocolate, and many people do, from time to time, try semisweet or dark chocolates. They have less saturated fat and their sharp flavor may let you feel more satisfied with less chocolate.

Here are some good rules of thumb for all sweets.

- Check out the fat content of all the sweets you eat—cookies, pastries, and other baked goods are usually dripping with fat. Find out how much fat is in a sweet, and if it contains more than 33 percent fat, choose again.

- Avoid low-fat versions of sweets if you can. The fat is usually replaced with sugar, and sugar can make you fat, too.

## JUNK-FOOD JUNKIE

*"My body is a temple where junk food goes to worship."*
—Anonymous

If you recorded eating 6 or more servings in this category in your food diary, chances are good that you are something of a Junk-Food Junkie. Don't worry, because you've got plenty of company. A recent study by Gladys Block at the University of California at Berkeley looked at the diet of just under 5,000 adults during 1999 and 2000. Block found that, on average, almost a third of the calories consumed by these individuals came from junk food.

A quarter of the calories we consume come from sweets, desserts, soda, and alcohol—foods with virtually no nutritional value and lots and lots of calories, the very definition of a junk food. When you add in chips and fruit drinks, you're up to 30 percent. Add in fast-food fare and you're consuming more than a third of your calories from what your mother would describe as junk food. The five foods that contribute the greatest number of calories to the American diet are: soda, pastries, hamburgers, pizza, and chips. All of these are foods that would be considered by most of us to be junk foods.

Although you might be surprised by the numbers, the facts behind them probably are no surprise to those of you who find yourself reading this section. A few years ago, writer Eric Schlosser tagged us as the Fast Food Nation. You and I know it's true. And we feel bad about it. How can we not when anti-obesity forces call for a "sin food tax." Eating these foods is now considered a sin. I'm not buying into that and you shouldn't either.

## Junk Food 101

First, let's define junk food so that we all know what we're talking about. When I say junk food, most of us will have a picture of what I mean: sodas, chips, fast-food fries. Most nutrition organizations define junk food as those foods that have a low nutrient/calorie ratio. That is to say, they deliver relatively few nutrients and lots of calories. Certainly, even a quick glance at the food label of many of our most popular junk foods will show that. Look at soda. A 20-ounce serving of Coca-Cola contains 250 calories and not much else. There are no vitamins, no minerals, no proteins. On the other hand, Coke contains no fats. The ingredients show that too. Coke is made from carbonated water, high-fructose corn syrup, phosphoric acid (a preservative), "natural flavors" (the secret recipe for Coke said to be kept in a safe in the Atlanta headquarters), and caffeine. Not much to go on nutrition-wise. And 250 calories. So a low nutrient/calorie ratio, for sure.

What about potato chips? Twenty chips is considered a serving (yeah, right). These twenty chips contain 150 calories of which 60 percent come from fats and 20 percent come from saturated fats. There's a dash of salt and a nearly accidental sprinkling of vitamin A, a couple of Bs, and a little C and E. Again, a low calorie-to-nutrient ratio. Although soda and chips are the favorite targets of those who seek to get them out of our diets, there are tons of foods that don't make it onto that list but are just as bad. Take that epitome of haute cuisine—pâté de foie gras. A serving size is listed as 1 tablespoon and contains 60 calories, 85 percent of which come from fat. There is a smidge of protein and again a practically accidental sprinkling of vitamins. So while pâté is not prominent on anyone's sin tax list, I'd put it in with the junk food as it's traditionally been defined. Same goes with many of the delicacies cherished by foodies everywhere. So let's get rid of the snobbery traditionally linked with the idea of junk food.

So now that we have defined our terms, let's look at what's known about these foods and obesity. You may guess that a diet high in these foods has been linked to obesity. Guess again. Despite the near-universal condemnation of junk food, the studies that have looked at the consumption of these foods haven't found a link. What they have found is that consumption of junk food is high in a large proportion of men, women, and children. No news there. But there is no correlation between the amount of junk food eaten and weight.

Skinny people eat junk food; overweight people eat junk food. Basically, most of us eat these foods, at least some of the time. So eating junk food does not make you fat.

There are some aspects of junk food eaters that are cause for concern. In the same studies that found no link between junk food and obesity, researchers did find that those who ate the most junk food often ate the least amount of fruits and vegetables. Eating fruits and vegetables won't necessarily make you thin (though it can't hurt), any more than eating junk food will make you fat, but these neglected foods do have components not found in junk foods and that are good for you: fiber, vitamins, minerals, and antioxidants. There is also good evidence that a diet high in fruits and veggies lowers your risk of high cholesterol, high blood pressure, and some cancers. A diet low in these foods increases your risk of lots of the chronic diseases that plague this country.

## The Case Against Soda

While the big category of junk food has not been linked to increased body weight, one very large component of the category has: soda. In studies done in children, teenagers, and adults, an increase in soda consumption is linked to a subsequent increase in weight. In a study done last year in *JAMA*, increasing soda consumption was also linked to a higher risk of developing diabetes. Why this is true is linked to the way our bodies measure calories. We have very finely controlled methods of measuring calorie intake built into our brains—we don't know how it works, but we know it's there. On average, we eat close to 1 million calories each year. Many people can do this without gaining a single pound and they can do it year after year after year. Yet an increase of one-tenth of 1 percent of our daily calories—the equivalent of ten M&Ms per day—would result in a weight gain of about 3–5 pounds per year. We aren't counting calories consciously, but our bodies are. Otherwise we would never be able to achieve the kind of perfect balance between what we eat and what we weigh. There are a couple of little loopholes in this otherwise very effective mechanism—and a big one is what we drink. Somehow, we don't register the calories we drink rather than eat. Measured at a single meal or over the long run, the calories we take in as fluids do not affect how much we eat or how many calories we take in. They just sneak right by our built-in calorie counter. So while most junk food may not be causing us to gain weight, there is good evidence that soft drinks, as well as other calorie-containing drinks, will.

If adding sodas can add weight, can eliminating sodas get rid of weight? Some studies suggest that very thing. In a recent study by Janet James featured in the *British Medical Journal*, schoolchildren who were encouraged to drink less soda did just that, and they lost weight. They weren't dieting, mind you, just drinking less soda. The researchers compared the class that was counseled to lose weight with another class that received no such counseling. Those kids drank more soda at the end of the year than they did at the start of the year and gained weight, too. Does this work in adults? The research here is a little less clear but some studies have shown this to be a successful strategy to minimize weight gain or lose weight.

## Junk Food—The Real Deal

You're here reading this chapter because you eat junk foods frequently. My job is to help you figure out some strategies for how to be able to work with the foods you love and still lose weight or maintain the weight you want. I think it can be done, even with these foods. My theory is that the difference between those who eat junk foods and have no difficulty managing their weight and those who do is not in what is eaten, but how it is eaten.

First, junk foods are often eaten when you are not hungry, and that's a pretty interesting phenomenon. There hasn't been a lot of research done in this area, but I'll share what has been done. Seeing food activates the whole brain. This occurs whether you are hungry or not. And the more palatable (scientific word for "tasty") the food you see, the stronger the urge to eat it—even if you are not hungry. The theory used to be that we eat in order to fill specific nutritional needs. It is clear that this is not the case. We eat because we are programmed to eat and we prefer foods that are high in salt, sugar, and fat. Hunger will make us seek food, but food itself will speak to us, even when we aren't hungry: The tastier the food, the louder the siren's song. It's no surprise then that what we call junk foods are going to be those most preferred when you are not hungry. They speak the loudest to us. They are among the most palatable foods made. Simply being around a stash of highly palatable foods can promote non-hunger eating.

One of the problems with eating when you are not hungry is that it doesn't change how much you eat when you get to your next meal. If you are hungry and you eat a snack, then when you get to your next meal, you will eat less food. Not so with snacks eaten when you are not hungry. Thus, foods eaten in the absence of hunger are just extra calories.

Although seeing palatable foods will increase the odds that many of us will eat them, not everyone does. Why that is true is still something of a mystery. It involves something called dietary restraint. For some people, seeing even highly palatable food when they are not hungry may be tempting, but they won't eat. Do these people simply have greater willpower? Maybe, but there is good evidence that some of this, perhaps most of this, is genetic. The children of adults with high levels of restraint also tend to have high levels of restraint. And the tendency to eat in the absence of hunger—a clear sign of low restraint—manifests itself at a very young age. It's been seen in children 4 and 5 years old—well before "bad habits" are really formed. So I think much of it is inborn. If you are one of those folks who can't resist a bowl of chips even after a big meal, blame it on your parents. Having said that, you need to work with who you are and try to avoid having these foods just lying around—even in cupboards. My daughter once told me that she was on a "see-food" diet—when she saw food she ate it. If you are one of those people, and I think it's a pretty common trait, then you need to make sure (to the extent you can) that you don't see it.

Another common way we eat junk food is when we are hungry—very hungry. Many marketing surveys have shown that people who eat at fast-food restaurants value the convenience of these restaurants. I suspect that is absolutely true. My own theory is that drive-through windows have done as much to our expanded waistlines as has "supersizing." When you are hungry, the call of the drive-through can be hard to ignore. You can keep driving and get home (or wherever you are going) and eat, or you could stop and eat now. Many choose now over later.

The real question is, why are you hungry? Here's why: We are designed to eat every few hours and yet we live our lives as if that were not the case. Many of us walk out of our houses each morning, knowing we won't be back until much later, but only a few have planned what to do between now and then about this completely predictable event. Like the chief of police in *Casablanca*, we are shocked, shocked I tell you, to find ourselves absolutely starving around lunchtime. At that point we look around to find something to eat and we certainly don't have to look far. But our ability to make a good choice at that point is very limited. In part we're limited by what's offered. Just as important, it's limited by our ability to make a knowledgeable choice. Few restaurants offer us nutritional data on the menu. (Ruby Tuesday—not a fast-food restaurant but a pretty big chain—now supplies nutritional info on each of their meals.) Fast-food restaurants have the data available but you usually can't get it in the restaurant, you have to get it from their Web site. You could avoid the fast-food restaurants altogether by simply bringing your lunch. It's a good idea and may make it easier to lose weight, but

I know that many people have enough to do each morning to fill several mornings and just don't have time to do that. But there are good choices to be made at any restaurant, even the fast-food restaurants. I have listed a few of these choices below. However, I would also recommend that you surf the net to find the fast-food restaurants near you and download their nutritional data. This way at least you know what you are getting, and knowledge is the start of power.

## Tips for Junk-Food Junkies, No Matter What Diet You Are On

1. Reduce the amount of calorie-laden drinks in your daily diet. If water has no appeal, try the flavored waters they are selling these days. Tea is another option. There is some evidence that teas (regular, not herbal teas) can help in weight loss.

2. Get rid of your home stashes of junk food. I know you tell yourself that they are for the kids but believe me, your kids can live without them—no matter what they might say. You home should be your haven against the onslaught of food that characterizes the world we live in today.

3. During the holiday season, when hightly palatable foods are everywhere, make sure you eat three meals a day and that you have a stash of healthy snacks available so that when you round a corner and confront a bowl of chocolate or a plate of freshly baked cookies, you at least have an option of running back to your desk and eating something that you like almost as much and which you will feel much better about eating.

4. If you can't bring your lunch and snacks to work, make sure you have a plan about what and where you will be eating when you get hungry. No plan means taking what comes— and that is probably part of what got you here in the first place.

5. If you find yourself starving and in a car, you can stop at a fast-food restaurant to eat. But think of that as a snack to

tide you over until you can eat something you will feel good about eating as a real meal. Below I have listed some possibilities and a few of the national chains. There are also several Web sites that let you look at all the foods from the chain restaurants. My favorite is www.foodfacts.info.

## FAST-FOOD FAVORITES

| Restaurant | Food | Calories | Fat (g) | Carbs (g) |
|---|---|---|---|---|
| Boston Market | ¼ rotisserie chicken | 280 | 12 | 2 |
| | ¼ rotisserie chicken, skin removed | 170 | 4 | 2 |
| | Honey-glazed ham | 210 | 8 | 10 |
| | Rotisserie turkey | 170 | 1 | 3 |
| Burger King | "Low carb" chicken Whopper (no bun, no mayo, ketchup) | 160 | 3.5 | 3 |
| | Veggie burger | 380 | 16 | 46 |
| | Salad (Caesar or garden) with chicken or shrimp (use a vinaigrette) | 200 | 10 | 13 |
| KFC | Original Recipe breast | 380 | 19 | 11 |
| | Original Recipe breast, skin removed | 140 | 3 | 0 |
| | Hot and spicy drumstick | 150 | 9 | 4 |
| | Cole slaw (½ cup) | 190 | 11 | 22 |
| | Corn on the cob (3 inches) | 70 | 1.5 | 13 |
| McDonald's | French fries (small) | 210 | 10 | 26 |
| | Milk shake, vanilla or strawberry | 420 | 10 | 72 |

|  |  |  |  |  |
|---|---|---|---|---|
|  | Chicken Select (3 pc) | 380 | 20 | 28 |
|  | Caesar, cobb, or bacon salad without chicken | 150 | 15 | 23 |
|  | Caesar, cobb, or bacon salad with chicken | 260 | 11 | 11 |
| Sonic | Grilled cheese | 282 | 12 | 39 |
|  | French fries | 195 | 11 | 22 |
|  | ChedR Peppers | 256 | 12 | 29 |
|  | Lemon slushy | 194 | 0 | 50 |
| Subway | 6-inch Veggie Delight | 230 | 3 | 44 |
|  | 6-inch roast beef, turkey, or ham | 290 | 5 | 47 |
| Taco Bell | Taco (order it salsa style to skip the cheese and dressing, and replace with salsa) | 170 | 9 | 12 |
| Wendy's | Small chili | 227 | 7 | 21 |
|  | Sour cream & chive potato | 370 | 5 | 73 |

# WATERLESS WONDER

*"With true friends . . . even water drunk together is sweet enough."* —Chinese proverb

If you listed 6 servings or fewer on question 7, there is a good chance you're not drinking enough.

When I first started keeping my own diet diary, I was shocked to see that on most days I drank only coffee with perhaps a glass of wine at the end of the day. Others have reported the same pattern.

The usual recommendation is that everyone should drink eight 8-ounce glasses of water each day. Most books on nutrition recommend this. What's the science behind this? Honestly, there isn't much. So what should a rational person do?

Let's start with the basics: Water is an essential nutrient. And we have only limited capabilities to store water. While our bodies are 70 percent water, that water is being used and is necessary. Moreover, we lose water every day. If we count only the water we lose by breathing and sweating—without even exercising—we lose 2 to 4 liters of water per day. That's not including urine or stools. Without water, the average person will die in 2 to 5 days, well before she would die from lack of food. So, water is essential, and, ultimately, more essential than food.

What is the optimal amount of water to drink when you are losing weight? Many diet books will tell you that drinking water helps flush fat and promotes weight loss. Maybe. There isn't any scientific literature on this, and you should know that anecdotal evidence is wrong at least as often as it is right.

When there is no data, opinion can flourish, so I'll give you my opinion. I think drinking a lot of water is good for you. I think it makes you feel better. I think it makes you look better and that your skin actually looks younger when you are well hydrated. And I think water consumption can contribute to weight loss. I'm not convinced that it helps "flush out" fat, except in the same sense that water flushes out much of our waste products.

I suspect that water consumption promotes weight loss, first, by contributing to our satiety (volume in the stomach helps to make you feel full) and, second, by helping us feel healthier. When we are clinically dehydrated, our bodies don't work well; physical performance can suffer when we lose as little as 1 to 2 pounds of water, and mental performance is measurably decreased when we lose 8 to 10 pounds of water. Mild to moderate dehydration has been linked to increased risk of bladder cancer (very rare in this country) and colon cancer (not so rare here).

So I say, drink up. Here's how you can tell if you are drinking enough water: Your urine should be very pale in color. If it's yellow or tan-colored, you aren't getting enough water.

If your heart is sinking at the prospect of drinking that much water, cheer up. Other fluids can provide the water you need plus some flavoring. Milk counts as a fluid; so do soft drinks. Juice counts as well. Even if you count those other drinks, chances are that you still fall short of your goal of eight glasses a day. How can you get all that water in?

I try to drink one 8-ounce glass of water every morning even before my coffee. Now I have a good start on my goal. And I try to drink one glass of water with every meal and snack. I frequently substitute either a soft drink (diet) or tea for water, especially with my snacks, and I try to squeeze in a glass of milk. One benefit I've noticed: I have developed a real love for plain cold water, especially first thing in the morning. On a good day I get to my target of eight glasses a day.

If you are exercising, you're going to need even more. Every year we get a news story about a young, extremely fit marine or football player who doesn't drink enough water. He or she gets overheated from too much exertion and gets carried off the field on a stretcher. If he's lucky, he survives. When you exercise, especially when it's hot, but at other times as well, drink before you play, drink as you play, and drink after you play. Your performance will be improved, and you will feel better.

Not everything that is served in a glass will count toward the magic goal of eight glasses per day. Below are a few brief descriptions of what we know about some of the different types of drinks in a normal American diet. "Beverage Pros and Cons" on page 283 summarizes these findings.

## What About Coffee?

*"The morning cup of coffee has an exhilaration about it which the cheering influence of the afternoon or evening cup of tea cannot be expected to reproduce."* —Oliver Wendell Holmes, Sr.

That exhilaration comes at least in part from the caffeine in the coffee, and caffeine is a mild diuretic. (A diuretic is a drug that promotes water loss, that is, it makes you pee.) So, you can't count on coffee to replace the water you lose.

Perhaps because of the caffeine and the exhilaration it produces, there is a sense that coffee is somehow bad for you and that tea is somehow good for you. This is a very old belief; researchers have been trying to pin down the truth for hundreds of years. The earliest controlled trial I have come across was actually conducted in eighteenth-century Sweden. A pair of identical twins had been sentenced to death for murder. King Gustave III thought that rather than execute these twins, he would put them to work in service to science. He spared the gallows-bound twins in return for their participation in a controlled trial of coffee drinking versus tea drinking. One twin had to drink three large bowls of tea every day, and his brother had to drink the same amount of coffee. The object was to see who lived longer.

Both outlived the curious king. But the tea drinker died first, at the ripe old age of 83. His coffee-consuming brother joined him in the graveyard just a couple of months later. I'm not sure that counts as a coffee victory.

But science has continued to consider this question. Here's what we know: Coffee increases blood pressure in those who drink it occasionally, although this doesn't appear to happen in habitual coffee drinkers. Coffee has been linked to elevated LDL cholesterol and other components that increase heart disease, but there is no evidence that coffee itself increases heart disease, despite many studies.

Researchers have tried, without much success, I must add, to link coffee to all kinds of awful health outcomes in addition to heart disease: miscarriages and cancer, mostly. So far none of these connections have been confirmed. It's thought that much of the apparent guilt of coffee is by association—due to lifestyle factors that often accompany coffee drinking, such as smoking. So, for now, coffee has a pretty clean bill of health.

Bottom line: Drink coffee if you enjoy it, but don't count it as a beverage when you are trying to determine whether or not you are getting enough to drink.

## How About Tea?

*"If you are cold, tea will warm you—if you are too heated, it will cool you—if you are depressed, it will cheer you—if you are excited, it will calm you."*—William Gladstone

Tea has always had a patina of virtue about it, the flip side to the dark aura of coffee. As it turns out, tea is full of antioxidants known as polyphenols and, at least in the laboratory, these ingredients have been shown to have effects that would reduce the risk of heart disease and cancer in humans. Does it pan out in the real world? It's not clear. Some studies have shown benefits to tea drinking; others have not. Tea drinking, like coffee drinking, has associated lifestyle factors that make measuring its effects more difficult.

By the way, when the virtues of tea are discussed, they are associated only with black tea, green tea, or oolong tea. All of these come from the leaves of the *Camellia sinensis*. The other types of infusions, which are often called herbal teas, don't really count as teas. And while they count toward your daily intake of liquids, they don't contain polyphenols.

I'm from the South, where you always have two iced tea choices: sweet tea or plain. And when they say sweet, they mean it. When you drink that sweet tea, Southern style, it might as well be a cola. That's okay in small quantities, but adding sugar to tea just increases its calories.

Bottom line: Drink tea if you enjoy it; it may even be good for you. Just don't load it up with sugar.

## What About Juice?

Let me reveal a prejudice here: I don't get juice drinking. I like the occasional V-8 juice and some homemade juices, but from my perspective, juice has lots of calories, little or no fiber, and only a touch of vitamins. If you ate the fruit itself rather than drinking the juice, you would get fewer calories, more fiber, and more vitamins. Plus you would feel fuller.

Can you have a glass of juice every now and then because you like it? Sure, but don't drink it because you think it's good for you. With very few exceptions, juice has about the same nutritional value as a soft drink.

Bottom line: Drink juices sparingly; if you love the taste, use a touch of them to flavor your water.

## How About Soft Drinks?

Obviously, soft drinks contain lots and lots of sugar. And lately they come in 20-ounce bottles and cups that you can practically bathe in, so it's very easy to overconsume them.

Here's something else about soft drinks: They can make you fat—and not just because they're loaded with calories. There is something else going on here. Over the past 20 years, soft drink manufacturers (and manufacturers of other sweet products as well) have stopped using cane sugar—you know, the white stuff that comes in a bag at the grocery store. They have replaced cane sugar with a sweetener made from corn. Corn sweeteners contain a type of sugar called fructose. In your body, fructose acts differently than glucose, the sugar most commonly found in your system. For example, glucose requires insulin in order to be taken up into cells. Fructose doesn't. Fructose also reduces circulating leptin levels. Both insulin and leptin play important roles in getting us to quit eating at the end of a meal or snack, so there is some concern that fructose is helping us get fat by allowing us to take in calories without feeling their filling effect. (It just goes to show you how complicated our bodies are—too much insulin can make you fat; it turns out that too little may also.)

Fructose consumption in test animals induces insulin resistance, impaired glucose tolerance, high blood pressure, and high triglyceride levels. The data in humans are less clear, although there is some evidence that it can affect us the same way it does mice. From my perspective, this is yet another reason to avoid soft drinks.

Bottom line: If you like soft drinks, you can drink them on occasion. If you can tolerate the switch to diet, drink that. If not, then think of a soft drink as a treat, like dessert, to be indulged in rarely and savored fully.

## What About Liquor, Wine, or Beer?

> *"Burgundy makes you think of silly things; Bordeaux makes you talk about them; and Champagne makes you do them."*
> —Jean-Anthelme Brillat-Savarin

Alcohols contain 7 calories per gram, almost twice what soft drinks have. So when you drink, you are loading up on calories. On the other hand, we rarely drink alcohol (except possibly beer) in the quantities that characterize how many of us drink soft drinks. So while alcohol contains lots of calories, that's probably not the most important way it contributes to our national waistline.

The more important problem with alcohol is that it lowers your inhibitions. It turns out your mother was right about this, too. It lowers your inhibitions about drinking more; it also lowers your inhibitions about eating more. Research has shown that drinking wine with meals causes people to stay longer at the table and to consume more food calories. A glass of wine with dinner is a pleasure, but just assume that when you drink with a meal, you will also eat more.

In addition, alcohol has some diuretic effects. One of the reasons (although not the only one) you feel so bad the day after you drink too much is that you are dehydrated. Drinking alcohol causes a net fluid loss, so it doesn't count toward your eight glasses a day.

On the other hand, alcohol has been shown to decrease the risk of heart disease. In a study of 38,000 American male doctors and dentists, men who drank moderately (between one and three glasses, five to seven nights a week) had a lower risk of heart disease than those who didn't drink at all. And—this is surprising—it didn't seem to matter whether they drank beer or liquor or wine.

Bottom line: Avoid alcohol when you are actively trying to lose weight; when your weight is stable, alcohol in moderation can improve your health. And because it's a diuretic, it doesn't count toward your eight-glass goal.

## Tips for Waterless Wonders, No Matter What Diet You Are On

**For carbohydrate counters:** Drinking your basic eight glasses of water a day is particularly important for you for two reasons. First, a diet low in carbs is high in proteins. No matter what you eat, you have to drink enough water to flush the waste out, and with proteins there is more waste. In order to deal with this, you will need to drink extra water.

The second reason is that constipation is a big complaint of many on this diet, at least in the early part. Water can help prevent constipation. Eight glasses will be enough; make sure you get that much water every day.

# BEVERAGE PROS AND CONS

| Drink | Pros | Cons | Bottom Line |
| --- | --- | --- | --- |
| Alcohol | Modest alcohol consumption improves cardiovascular risk factors | Contains 7 calories per gram; lowers inhibitions, which promotes overeating | Avoid alcohol while actively trying to lose weight. Limit alcohol intake to one (women) or two (men) drinks per night to maximize benefits and reduce risks. Does not count toward your eight glasses. |
| Coffee | A good medium for milk | Caffeine is a diuretic | Caffeinated coffee doesn't count toward your eight glasses. |
| Herbal Tea | Has no caffeine | Often gets loaded with sugar | Counts toward your eight glasses |
| Milk | Promotes bone growth and weight loss | Contains lots of saturated fats and carbohydrates | Drink fat-free or 1% milk to reduce the amount of fat in your diet. Counts toward your eight glasses. |
| Tea | Has antioxidants in it; has much less caffeine than coffee | Often gets loaded with sugar | Counts toward your eight glasses |

| Soft Drinks | Contain lots of water | Contain lots of sugar; may promote weight gain | Drink diet soft drinks to reduce intake. Count toward your eight glasses. |
|---|---|---|---|

**For calorie counters:** You will be taking in more protein as you cut calories, so make sure you get enough water to flush out the waste products left over after you use the proteins. Watch your urine, and if it looks darker than water, you need to drink more liquids.

**For fat counters:** You will be eating foods that have a very high water content, so your need for extra liquid is lower than those on the other types of diets. Still, you need to monitor your urine. If it looks darker than water, increase the amount of water you drink.

## PROP TASTER

*"An onion can make people cry, but there has never been a vegetable invented to make them laugh."*
—Will Rogers (a suspected PROP taster)

If you scored 40 or higher on the PROP test, chances are that you are what is known as a taster, and if you scored higher than 80, you may even be a supertaster.

PROP is a naturally occurring chemical in food; its only real importance lies in its ability to identify those of us which are sensitive to the bitter flavors of some foods—particularly vegetables. If you can taste it, you are genetically programmed to dislike important and health-promoting foods such as broccoli, spinach, brussels sprouts, cabbage, and grapefruit because of their bitterness. As it turns out, liking these vegetables and fruits may be a rare quality. Up to 75 percent of the world's population are PROP tasters and a mere 25 percent nontasters, that is, folks who are insensitive to the bitterness of PROP and many of the foods that are so good for you.

When researchers have studied tasters and supertasters, they have found that, in general, both groups dislike brussels sprouts, cauliflower, cabbage, radishes, and grapefruit more than nontasters. Other foods disliked by tasters include coffee, green tea, and bitter beers. In addition, the group described as supertasters tend to dislike foods that are very sweet or that have a high fat content. This makes supertasters perhaps the pickiest eaters in the world.

Is there an association between your PROP-taster status and weight? It makes sense, but so far the studies are not conclusive. In some surveys, supertasters were thinner than nontasters. Why would they be thinner? Since supertasters have many more food aversions than nontasters, it is possible that they eat a very bland, unvaried diet, and diets with less variety have been associated with a lower BMI.

If how things taste is determined by your genes, you can't be blamed for not eating your broccoli. Doctors and nutritionists have insisted that we all should eat a diet low in fat and high in fruits and vegetables. The fact that these foods don't taste good to a significant portion of the population hasn't really even been discussed.

The genetic basis of taste is not a new discovery. In the 1930s, a chemist named A. L. Fox was working with a chemical very similar to PROP, and some of it accidentally became airborne. Fox's colleague immediately noted and commented on the bitter taste of the airborne stuff, but Fox himself tasted nothing. That simple observation led to hundreds of family studies investigating the genetic varieties in the ability to taste PROP.

Since then, populations across the globe have been tested for this trait. In western Africa, 97 percent of the population are tasters. In India, only 60 percent are. In the adult population of the United States, 75 percent are tasters. In general, the ability to taste PROP is strongest when you are younger and declines slowly with age. It's more common in women than men. In women, the ability to taste PROP is influenced by sex hormones, so it fluctuates over the course of the menstrual cycle and in pregnancy.

Although exactly how this trait works is not well understood, there are measurable differences between tasters, nontasters, and supertasters. For one thing, tasters have more taste buds than nontasters, and supertasters have even more than tasters. And some researchers have found that there are different sensitivities to different types of bitterness even among tasters—that some of us may be more sensitive to the taste of quinine; others, to the taste of PROP. Current thinking is that there may be up to sixty different receptors just for the perception of bitterness.

This is an active area of research, simply because what we eat is important and many of the foods currently thought of as good for us (such as fruits and vegetables) are not widely consumed despite active encouragement. The reason doctors and nutritionists want you to eat these fruits and vegetables is that they contain disease-reducing chemicals that can help you stay healthy longer. In a number of population-based studies like the Harvard Nurses' Study, higher consumption of fruits and vegetables was associated with lower rates of many cancers as well as lower rates of obesity and heart disease.

The goal of this research is to see if there is a biological and genetic reason for our eating habits and then try to fix it. So, if you hate broccoli, as did former president George Bush *père,* consider that this may be inherited. You can't help it if you don't like it; you got it from your mom or dad. On the other hand, research also indicates that sensitivity to bitterness is highest in young children, and this is the age when food preferences are determined. It is possible that the vegetable you hated as a child will taste pretty good now, but first you have to taste it.

The other thing to do, since fruits and vegetables are an important part of a diet and grossly underconsumed, is to actively look for ones you like. Too often, we are introduced to only a few vegetables before our mothers throw up their hands in despair and give up. We generalize from our experience with broccoli and spinach that we do not like vegetables. Let me encourage you to try other (nonbitter) vegetables and fruits. (A list of nonbitter vegetables is provided on page 288.) We live in a world where we can eat just about everything. Use this ability to expand your horizons vegetable-wise.

## Tips for PROP Tasters, No Matter What Diet You Are On

1. Eat the youngest leaves of leafy greens. Often young leaves have much less of the bitter flavor than more mature leaves.

2. Cook bitter vegetables in ways that reduce their bitter flavors. The most common way is to cook the vegetable at a high heat in a little olive oil with garlic. Or use 1 to 2 tablespoons of olive oil and ¼ to ½ cup fat-free chicken broth or white wine. Simmer until tender.

3. Salt decreases bitterness. Season bitter vegetables generously with salt and see if you like them more.

4. Combine vegetables with starches. This is a common practice in Italian foods where bitter greens are mixed with bland white beans or pastas to make them more palatable. It's one way to use the tang of the vegetables to liven up the smooth blandness of the starch.

5. Use small amounts of vegetables as ingredients in other dishes. This way you will increase your vegetable intake in an enjoyable way. Broccoli or spinach quiche is a classic example. There are others out there. Just look around.

6. Very few fruits have bitter flavors. Grapefruit is probably the worst. Other exceptions are rhubarb and persimmons. So if you can't get yourself past your loathing of vegetables, try to increase your intake of fruits from the wide variety nature offers.

## NONBITTER VEGETABLES FOR PROP TASTERS

(The foods in **bold print** are best for the 30-gram Counting Carbohydrates Diet; all are acceptable on the 100-gram Counting Carbohydrates Diet.)

| | |
|---|---|
| **Artichoke** | Lentils |
| **Asparagus** | **Lettuce (many varieties)** |
| **Avocado** | **Mushrooms** |
| Beans—virtually all varieties | Okra |
| Beets | **Olives** |
| Carrots | Parsnips |
| **Celery** | Peas |
| Chickpeas | Potatoes |
| Corn | Pumpkin |
| **Cucumbers** | **Soybeans, green (edamame)** |
| Eggplant | Squash |
| Green peppers | Sweet potatoes |
| **Hot peppers** | **Tomatoes** |
| Jicama | Turnips |
| **Leeks** | Yams |

**For carbohydrate counters:** One of the easiest ways to reduce the bitterness of many vegetables is to add salt and butter. While butter is nothing but saturated fat, and filled with calories, the benefit it offers in making these important foods palatable outweighs the downside, especially on this diet. So, as you are cooking, feel free to use a modest amount of butter to enhance the taste of vegetables, if that makes them more appealing.

You'll also find that many of these vegetables taste wonderful in a casserole made with eggs and cheese. Recipes for this type of casserole abound in cookbooks and on the Web.

**For calorie counters:** Most of these foods are wonderfully low in calories, so you can combine them with other foods to make them more palatable. Mixing greens or other bitter vegetables with a starch is a classic way of improving on both the tang of the vegetable and the blandness of the starch. Normally, bitter greens such as spinach and collards can be sautéed in oil and broth or wine and then added to a pasta for a different taste. Including these foods in your diet will increase your variety without increasing your calorie count, so try it; you'll like it.

**For fat counters:** Since fruits and vegetables will make up the bulk (literally) of what you eat, it's very important to expand your horizons if you are a PROP taster. In addition to trying new foods, try new ways of preparing the same old stuff. Asian cuisines— Indian, Thai, Chinese, Japanese—offer a variety of ways to cook these foods to minimize the bitterness that may be there. If you like them, you should invest in one or two good cookbooks to give you more ways to prepare these essential foods. A touch of exotic oil like walnut oil or sesame oil can bring new life and flavors to the same old dishes, and I encourage you to try some.

# CHAPTER 10
## DIETING HISTORY

### VOLUME

*"My doctor told me to stop having intimate dinners for four. Unless there are three other people."* —Orson Welles

If you selected mostly *a*'s in the What Makes You Feel Full section of the questionnaire, then one of the cues telling you that you have eaten enough is volume. There are two aspects of volume: The first is visually determined and at least partially psychological. When you look at your plate, you think, This is (or is not) enough food to satisfy me. Your assessment, which is based on how much it has previously taken to fill you, creates an expectation of satiety. The second aspect of volume is physiological: You eat a certain amount of food, and it fills you up—literally.

Let's talk about the visual cues first. One of the things I hear from my patients is that they sometimes have a sense when they are dieting that the amount of food they're eating simply isn't enough. They look at the recommended portion of meat—the size of their palm—and think, This can't possibly be enough to fill me up. They know how much they normally eat, and that is not it.

It may have come as a surprise to you to hear that the judgment about what constitutes a normal-size portion is learned. It is based on how much you have eaten as a portion in the past. This learned response can change, and has changed a lot in recent decades. Over the past 25 years or so, thanks to the success of a guy named David Wallerstein, serving size has increased dramatically. Wallerstein (whose dubious achievement was recently described in the terrific book about the fattening of America, *Fat Land*, by Greg Critser) was trying to increase profits at a chain of movie theaters by getting theatergoers to buy more popcorn. But try as he might, he couldn't induce people to buy two bags. So he made larger single bags, and supersizing was born. It may not surprise you to hear that Wallerstein is now an executive at McDonald's.

Although supersizing is specific to fast-food places, the idea that you can make a lot more money by offering people a lot more food has permeated our society at every level. From candy bars to the foods served in our finest restaurants, portion size has gone up, up, up. Nouvelle cuisine was a phenomenon in the 1990s, for those of you too young to remember. The coup de grâce of this short-lived fad was the feeling that you didn't get enough food for the money when eating these beautiful but spare meals. No restaurateur has made that mistake since, you can be sure of that.

Marketers and researchers have demonstrated that portion size—that is, how much we think it will take to make us full—is learned and can change based on what is available. When presented with larger portions, people will eat up to 30 percent more than they otherwise would. Human hunger is apparently quite elastic, which makes excellent evolutionary sense: Our hunter-gatherer ancestors ate whenever the eating was good, thereby storing reserves of fat against future famine. The problem is that in an era of abundance, the opportunity for feasting now presents itself 24/7—and at bargain prices.

Researchers in Sweden recruited twenty-seven subjects, overweight and normal weight, and had them eat a meal on two separate occasions. Before each meal, they were asked how hungry they were, and after each meal, they were asked how satisfied they were. The first meal was a normal meal, and the second meal was eaten blindfolded. When blindfolded, the participants ate 20 percent less of the same meal than they did when they could see the food. Seeing the food drove the participants to eat what they thought was their normal serving, even though less food would have been just as satisfying.

So, for those who have a strong visual component to their sense of fullness, know that it is adjustable in a way that other types of satiety are not.

The other kind of satisfaction provided by volume is the feeling that comes from your gastrointestinal tract. As researcher Barbara Rolls, Ph.D., demonstrated, many of us tend to eat the same volume of food, regardless of the calorie count. Here's how her research has been done. She recruits a group of volunteers—she's done these types of experiments on both normal weight and overweight folks—and she will feed these volunteers one or more meals in a given day. Then she asks them to write down everything they eat for the rest of that day. Each volunteer will do this several times over the course of the experiment. What the volunteers do not know is that, although the meals she prepares for them all look and taste similar, they have different amounts of calories: One meal might have a lot of calories; the next, fewer. They eat and then record everything else they eat and drink for the next day or so after the meal. Typically, these studies last only a couple of days, but several have followed food amounts for up to 11 weeks.

Here's what Dr. Rolls discovered: Most people ate the same amount of food independent of the calories in the meal. That is, whether the meal was mostly pasta (lots of calories) or mostly veggies (fewer calories), the volunteers ate the same volume of food in all the meals. And they didn't overeat later to compensate. Based on their food diaries, on days when the research meal was low in calories, they just ate fewer calories. Their level of hunger and satisfaction were the same. Thus, researchers concluded that for many of us, volume is a more important aspect of satisfaction than calorie content.

If you're one of these people, you can fill yourself with low-calorie foods and feel just as full and satisfied as if you had eaten high-calorie foods. If so, you are most likely to do well on a low-fat diet that emphasizes the replacement of high-calorie fats with low-calorie carbohydrates.

Even within the category of carbohydrates, you can replace high-calorie carbs—pasta, rice, cakes, and cookies—with low-calorie substitutes like vegetables and fruits. You don't eliminate the pasta, but you replace some of it with a lower-calorie substitute, and you end up eating fewer calories but still feeling full.

Although those who depend on volume for satiety do well on the Counting Fats Diet, this principle will work with just about any other diet, too.

## Tips for Those Who Need Volume, No Matter What Diet They Are On

1. Use fruits and vegetables as volume providers. Think of your plate as a pie chart; fill half of the plate with your fruits or vegetables, and the other half should be evenly divided between the meat and the starch.

2. Recalibrate your visual sense of what a serving is. To do this, measure all of your portions, at least for the first 2 weeks. Learn what a ½-cup serving looks like on a plate. Our expectations of what 1 serving is has crept up along with our weight.

3. Serve yourself food one portion at a time. Research has shown that the larger the serving, the more we eat. Four ounces of meat may not seem like much, because our sense of portion is so out of whack, but it may fill you up. If it doesn't, you can always go back for seconds.

4. Don't buy economy-size anything. Studies have shown that the amount of food you expect to eat as a single portion increases as the size of the container it comes from increases.

**For carbohydrate counters:** The temptation for you is going to be to eat more protein and fat rather than carbohydrates in your search for more food. Don't do it. Serve yourself some more salad or vegetables and, if you are still hungry, consider seconds of the meat. If you really need volume to feel full, vegetables provide more bulk and volume than meat.

A rule of thumb: If you still feel hungry right after you have eaten your meal, then you may need more volume. When that happens, eat more vegetables. If you feel full after you eat but get hungry again after an hour or two, then increase the size of your protein portion.

**For calorie counters:** Use high-calorie foods as flavorings for low-calorie foods. Your chili should be more beans than meat; your stew should be more potatoes, carrots, onions, and peas than meat. Strawberry shortcake should be heavy on the strawberries and light on the shortcake and whipped cream.

**For fat counters:** Combine starches with lower-calorie carbohydrates. When you make pasta or rice, add vegetables for flavor and volume.

# VARIETY

*"VARIETY is the soul of pleasure."* —Aphra Behn

If you found yourself checking mostly *b*'s in the What Makes You Feel Full section, then you depend on variety to make you feel full and satisfied. The hardwired drive to crave a variety of foods makes itself felt at a very early age. Studies show that children as young as 3 years old will choose a diet composed of a variety of foods even if they've been offered a favorite food.

Researchers in England first noted in rhesus monkeys that the pleasure associated with any given food decreases as the food is eaten. And that was true even if the offered food was a favorite. After a relatively short while, the pleasure afforded by that food diminished enough so that the desire for other foods was stronger, and the monkeys stopped eating one food and started on another. The researcher named this phenomenon "sensory-specific satiety."

As it turns out, humans work the same way. A food, no matter how loved, will lose some of its pleasure-giving power as soon as it is eaten so that other foods, even those less desirable, become more preferred. This is because variety offers us the best chance for obtaining all the nutrients essential in life.

If variety promotes eating more, then limiting variety ought to make it easier to eat less and easier to lose weight. This is certainly how many diets work. And it does work—for a while. But can you limit your food choices forever? I think some people can. We all know people who eat virtually the same foods day after day after day and seem to enjoy that. But for most of us, food choices are driven at least in part by a need for variety.

Many people have told me that one reason they found diets so hard to stick to is the limitation on the selection of foods. One of the greatest attributes of Weight Watchers is that, although it rewards a low-fat, low-calorie diet, *nothing* is forbidden. Variety is allowed, even encouraged. And Weight Watchers is at least as successful as other weight-loss programs.

How is it possible for variety to promote obesity but also be used successfully in weight loss? Because the drive for variety resides in your mouth, and since this drive for any given food is quickly satisfied, we, like the monkeys, can move on to the next food.

So, if you crave variety in your diet, then you can harness that to help you eat less food by eating a wider variety at each meal. But—and this is key—you must limit your portions so that you don't end up increasing your variety *and* the amount of food. If you can learn to enjoy a small portion of a wide variety of foods, this can be a successful strategy for losing weight. In fact, in my Counting Fats and Counting Calories diets, I offer small portions of several foods at each meal to try to harness the power of variety and improve satisfaction despite limiting calories.

## Tips for Those Who Need Variety, No Matter What Diet They Are On

1. Incorporate variety into all your meals. The temptation is to just eat a lot of a single food—a bowl of cereal in the morning; the same green salad at lunch. Don't do it. It is more work, but you will find it easier to eat less overall if at every meal you include different food types and textures. Don't save that for dinnertime when you have more time but are more likely to overeat.

2. When you eat out, order a couple of appetizers and skip the entrée.

3. With every meal try to have foods that are different in several ways. Have something crunchy, something smooth, something cool and refreshing, something spicy.

4. One easy way to increase variety is to add a low-calorie soup to your menu.

5. Sweets are also part of the variety we crave. Try incorporating a small serving of fruits or a low-calorie sweet into most of your meals. This may also reduce your risk of bingeing on sweets (for those of you who have this tendency).

6. Identify your cravings and incorporate that food (or a key aspect of that food) into your next meal or snack. If you find yourself craving a slice of cake, try to figure out what it is that appeals to you about that right then. Is it a desire for something sweet? Then have some fruit or maybe a piece of gum. Is it something smooth that you want? Have low-fat yogurt or a low-fat ice cream sandwich. Something buttery? Try a piece of toast sprayed with butter. By isolating the quality of the food you crave, you can try to satisfy it with a food that is lower in calories.

7. Remember, what you crave is variety, and your mouth can't tell how much of a food you are eating. Eat a small amount and see if that satisfies you. It often will.

8. The stronger the flavor of a food, the more rapidly we become sated with it and can move on to another flavor. This may be part of the reason bland-tasting "junk foods" or other carbohydrates are so easy to overeat. Many contain lots of calories and lots of fat but not so much flavor, so that the food doesn't trigger the signal that you've had enough. If you use variety to tell you when you have had enough, make sure that the foods you eat are flavorful and really speak to your taste buds. That's the key to this kind of satiety.

**For carbohydrate counters:** This type of diet is a real challenge for variety seekers, because at least part of its power comes from the limitation on variety. Even though your selection of foods is very restricted, especially in the early part of the diet, focus on providing yourself with a variety of textures and other sensory aspects of the food.

**For calorie counters:** This type of diet is really perfect for variety seekers because you can choose any type of food you want. The key for you is going to be portion control. If you don't get the variety you crave, you may still not feel satisfied. You might blame the small portions, but the real problem is insufficient variety or foods too bland to be counted. If you want to use variety to help you feel more full and satisfied with less food, choose foods that have a strong and enjoyable flavor.

**For fat counters:** Carbohydrates are naturally the most diverse of all food groups, so satisfying your need for variety should be relatively easy. Remember to serve yourself small portions, and if you are not satisfied at the end of the meal, consider trying a small portion of another low-calorie food rather than going back for seconds of foods you have already eaten.

## RICHNESS

*"I come from a family where gravy is considered a beverage."*
—Erma Bombeck

If you selected primarily *c*'s under What Makes You Feel Full on the questionnaire, then you respond to the composition of your meals rather than to their size or variety. In general, folks like you need to eat meat or some other source of protein to really feel full. You could eat a small steak and feel more full than if you ate a huge salad.

How this works still is not clear, but let me tell you what is known at this point. As background, you need to know that most meals are made up of a combination of carbohydrates, proteins, and fats. These comprise what is known as the macronutrient content of food (as opposed to the micronutrient content: vitamins and minerals). Research suggests that each of these three macronutrients has a different ability to reduce hunger.

Protein has been shown to have the greatest ability to reduce hunger. Carbohydrates are next. And fats do very poorly in reducing hunger; they help mainly by making the sensation of fullness last longer. How does this work? As soon as you put food in your mouth, your body is hard at work trying to break the food down into basic components that can then be absorbed into your bloodstream. There are enzymes in your mouth, which start breaking down simple carbohydrates. This is why you can get a sugary taste when you chew saltines for a long time; the amylase in your saliva breaks the cracker carbohydrate down to its most basic component, glucose, while it's still in your mouth. In your stomach and small intestines, enzymes go to work breaking down proteins and fats, and as these are absorbed, your body releases other chemicals to help process the foods.

## ONE-SERVING SNACKS

| Nuts or Seeds | Fat (g) | Calories | Carbohydrate (g) |
|---|---|---|---|
| Almonds, 1 oz (24 nuts) | 14 | 164 | 6 |
| Cashews, 1 oz (¼ cup) | 13 | 170 | 8 |
| Peanuts, 1 oz (¼ cup) | 14 | 180 | 6 |
| Pepitas, 1 oz (120 seeds) | 2 | 127 | 5 |
| Pine nuts, ¼ cup | 14 | 150 | 3 |
| Pistachios, 1 oz (45 nuts) | 12 | 155 | 3 |

## CARB/PROTEIN SNACK COMBINATIONS

| Snack | Fat (g) | Calories |
|---|---|---|
| Apple and low-fat string cheese | 5.5 | 145 |
| Carrots, celery, and 4 tbsp hummus | 6 | 140 |
| Celery stuffed with 1 tbsp cream cheese | 10 | 140 |
| Cucumbers, sliced, and ½ cup low-fat cottage cheese | 2 | 100 |
| Figs (2) and 1 oz prosciutto | 5 | 165 |
| Fruit Smoothie, small (½ recipe from page 177) | 2 | 155 |

| | | |
|---|---|---|
| Potato, baked, small, with 2 tbsp low-fat sour cream and salsa | 4 | 205 |
| Strawberries with 8 oz low-fat plain yogurt | 4 | 190 |
| Tortilla chips, baked, 20 chips, and Pico de Gallo (page 221) | 4 | 240 |

There is a multitude of these organic chemicals released, but the two most important are cholecystokinin (known as CCK) and insulin. CCK is specifically released in response to the consumption of proteins and fats, and insulin is specifically released in response to proteins and carbohydrates. These two chemicals work with the body to let you know when you have had enough to eat.

How? Well, CCK promotes a feeling of fullness by slowing down the rate at which the stomach moves food into the small intestine. Decreasing that rate keeps food in the stomach longer and allows a larger quantity of food to accumulate in the stomach. More food in the stomach is a signal that you have eaten enough. In addition, both CCK and insulin talk directly to the brain to let it know that the right amount of food has been eaten and that it's time to stop eating.

People who respond most strongly to this signal tend to do well on diets that emphasize proteins—either a calorie-counting diet or a carbohydrate-counting diet—because it is easier for them to eat less food overall if they eat more of the foods that make them feel full fastest.

## Tips for Those Who Need Richness, No Matter What Diet They Are On

1. Proteins and fats are very sating foods, so serving sizes can be modest.

2. Carbohydrates should always be eaten with a protein in order to help you feel full. I have listed several snacks on page

299 that combine carbs with a protein for a low-fat snack. Most of these snacks have 200 or fewer calories.

3. Those of you who need fat and protein to feel full may want to add nuts to the list of foods you can eat. They are rich in fats and protein, and they are good for you, too. But it's easy to overeat nuts. On page 299 are the amounts of nuts that make up a snack. I suggest you prepackage them in 1-serving helpings. That way, if you overeat, at least you are aware of it.

**For fat and calorie counters:** Remember that meat is not the only source of protein in a diet; eggs, dairy products, and many vegetables also contain large amounts of protein and should be a major component of your diet, since you need protein to feel full. Plan to make one or two meals a week vegetarian so that you can maintain a moderate fat intake on a weekly basis. *The Greens Cookbook* by Deborah Madison, my favorite vegetarian cookbook, has a wealth of recipes that provide good alternatives to meat as the meal's centerpiece. Also consider cookbooks from cultures with a heavily vegetarian population.

## DIETING BEHAVIOR

If you had a score greater than 30 in the How Dieting Changes the Way You Eat section, then you may have dieting behaviors that contribute to your inability to control your weight.

Psychiatrists have identified three attributes of eating behavior that affect dieters' ability to lose weight and keep it off. The three qualities are:

1. Dietary restraint—the extent to which you try to select foods that are consistent with your dietary goal and reject foods that are not. This is, for example, choosing fruit for dessert rather than a slice of chocolate cake. You allow yourself a dessert, but one that you know has fewer calories.

2. Hunger—your perception of your need for food.

3. Disinhibition—the extent to which you eat, or possibly overeat, in response to the presence of yummy food or other stimuli, such as emotional distress. For example, Judy craves cookies when she gets angry or annoyed at work. When she really wants to yell at someone, she often finds herself at the snack machine scarfing down cookies.

Having restraint makes it easier to lose weight or maintain that new weight. Disinhibition makes both harder—this may seem pretty obvious. But it's actually a little more complicated than that. Many dieters who have high restraint can also have high levels of disinhibition. In fact, this seems to be a particularly common combination in yo-yo dieters. Here is how it works: A high level of restraint is often associated with very rigid attitudes about eating. When something prevents the dieter from eating exactly as she plans, her dietary restraint breaks down, and her disinhibition leads her to eat in a way that is completely *counter* to her ideals.

This can sometimes even lead to episodes of bingeing. In other words, if you end up at McDonald's—because you're traveling and arrived after other places had closed or because you were late and didn't have a chance to eat but now you just want to grab something quick—you're upset because you're breaking your diet. Because you're upset, you're tempted to overeat once you are there.

What can you do if you have a high level of disinhibition? Awareness is important but not sufficient. In general, the best strategy is to figure out what your triggers are and either avoid them or come up with an alternate plan to the usual eating response. For those dieters who have high levels of restraint and high levels of disinhibition, the goal should be to develop some flexibility in how you think about your diet. When you eat something that is not on your diet (which is inevitable—no one is perfect), you need to be careful of how you handle that. The temptation is to say, "Well, now that I have erred, what the hell. I'll start the diet again tomorrow," and then eat in a disinhibited way. A better alternative is to think, Well, I screwed up. Let's try to get back on track, starting now. You need to recognize that the error was not necessarily in eating what you ate, but in the decisions that made that eating possible. Did you forget to pack a lunch? Did you have to go on a trip unexpectedly and end up missing breakfast, lunch, or dinner? Figure out what led to your aberration and learn to recognize that pattern. Your chances of minimizing future errors will be greatly enhanced.

It's easier said than done, as you know. But recognizing these behaviors and working to change them is essential to successful weight-loss maintenance.

## BINGE EATING DISORDER

*"Life itself is the proper binge."* —Julia Child

If you scored 11 or higher on this section, you may have binge eating disorder. Doctors increasingly recognize that a small but significant minority of overweight individuals struggle with episodes of massive overeating. Overeaters Anonymous popularized the most widely used term for this—compulsive overeating. Psychiatrists call this binge eating disorder.

This disorder is characterized by episodes of uncontrolled eating during which the individual feels that she has lost control of her ability to stop. She may eat large quantities of food and not stop until she feels uncomfortably, painfully full. These individuals may binge frequently—as much as twice a week and often more. Frequently these binges occur when alone, and an episode of bingeing is often followed by feelings of guilt and self-loathing. Obviously, individuals with this disorder have more difficulty losing weight and keeping it off. Many of them are obese and have a history of weight fluctuations.

There is a variation of binge eating that has been recently recognized, called night eating syndrome. In this disorder, individuals consume more than 50 percent of their total caloric intake at night, often eating when they are unable to fall asleep or even waking up at night and bingeing before going back to bed. If you think that you may have one of these disorders, do yourself a big favor and talk to your physician about it. The presence of these problems makes losing weight particularly difficult.

Many people with binge eating disorder can be helped through talk therapy or structured weight-loss programs that address their particular needs. Overeaters Anonymous is recommended by many experts in the field, although there is no published data on this group's success rate. You need to recognize this problem and find the assistance you need in order to manage your weight.

# CHAPTER 11
## MEDICAL HISTORY

THE MOST IMPORTANT REASON for changing your diet and losing weight is to help you become healthier. Of course, even though the majority of Americans are trying to lose weight, the goal, far too often, is simply to look good. Luckily, so long as you choose a reasonable diet, the health benefits are automatic.

In fact, you don't even have to lose weight to see many of the benefits from what we think of as dieting. Simply choosing your food carefully and increasing your activity level—those things that most of us mean when we say we are on a diet—can dramatically improve your health and lengthen your life. When you actually lose weight and bring yourself closer to a BMI of under 26, the health benefits really start to roll in.

A 10-percent weight loss will go a long way toward fixing what ails you. It will bring down your blood pressure (if it's too high), reduce your cholesterol, improve your blood sugar and insulin, and reduce your risk of developing diabetes or heart disease.

Your target weight is a personal decision based on how you want to look and feel, and I can't tell you what you should weigh. This much I can tell you, though: A loss of 5 to 10 percent of your weight will help you feel better, be healthier, and live longer. When people say that diets don't work, they are talking about how hard it is for many, and maybe for most, of us to reach what we feel is our ideal weight. But, even if you never achieve that elusive goal, the one way that diets can work is by making you healthier.

On the other hand, many of us have at least one health problem that can be improved by how we eat, and that is what this chapter is all about. I've tried to condense this important information to make it as accessible as possible, to give you concrete suggestions on modifying your diet to address your health needs as you lose weight. But, of course, before you start on this (or any) diet program, you should consult your doctor. Successful weight loss will have an effect on many health problems, and you may need to adjust your medications as you progress toward your goal.

## YOUR MEDICAL HISTORY

If you have a score of 3 or greater in this section of the questionnaire, then you may be at increased risk of developing heart disease. In general, cardiac risk factors are divided into those that are modifiable (those that have to do with lifestyle and the development and treatment of chronic disease) and those that are not (primarily sex and age).

In general, older individuals are at higher risk than younger, and men are at risk at a younger age than women. You can't do much about these factors, so let's move on to those you can influence. In this section, I will tell you what the research shows that you should be eating if you have any of these underlying medical conditions.

## SMOKING

Not exactly news to anyone, but smoking is bad for you. What may surprise you, however, is that most smokers don't die of lung cancer or emphysema. The vast majority of smokers die from heart disease.

A common reason for not quitting smoking is fear of weight gain. The average amount of weight gained during smoking cessation is 6 pounds. On the other hand, once you quit smoking it's easier to lose weight, because it's easier to live an active life, and that helps with weight loss.

It is hard to quit. (I quit after smoking for 15 years, and I still consider that to be one of the great achievements of my life.) But it can be done. Research suggests that the use of a nicotine-replacement device—either the patch, the inhaler, the gum, or the candy—plus the use of Wellbutrin SR starting 1 to 2 weeks prior to quitting is a pretty successful combo.

Those of you who aren't yet able to quit (I wouldn't be much of a doctor if I didn't think there was always hope) should address the other cardiac risk factors that place you at higher risk. Below I've listed some of the ways diet can help you with this.

In addition, smokers as well as former smokers may be able to reduce their risk of developing lung cancer by eating a diet high in fruits and vegetables. In some studies, smokers who ate a diet rich in fruits and vegetables (more than 5 servings per day) decreased their risk of lung cancer by a third.

You might be tempted to skip the fruits and vegetables and just take beta-carotene, vitamin E, or other antioxidants in pill form.

Don't do it. When studies compared smokers who took these supplements with those who did not, taking the antioxidants actually increased the cancer risk, rather than reducing it. And in participants who ate lots of fruits and veggies and took antioxidants, the two interventions cancelled each other out—so they were at the same risk as those who did neither.

A diet rich in omega fats may also reduce your risk of lung cancer and heart disease. In a study done in Greece (which has one of the highest rates of smoking in the world), men who ate the traditional Mediterranean diet—rich in fruits, vegetables, and fish—lived much longer than those who did not.

Bottom line: Quitting smoking is the most effective way to improve your health. Even if you can't quit (yet), a diet high in fruits, vegetables, and seafood will reduce your risk of dying from smoking-related heart disease and cancer.

## CHOLESTEROL

As you probably know by now, there are several different types of cholesterol that should be measured by your doctor. A quick refresher about each of them. First, there is the so-called bad cholesterol, LDL. This is the form of cholesterol most highly correlated with risk of heart attack or stroke. Healthy people should have an LDL cholesterol level of less than 160 milligrams per deciliter (mg/dl). People who either have diabetes or have had heart disease in the past and so are at a higher risk of heart disease should have an LDL cholesterol level of less than 70 mg/dl.

HDL cholesterol is the so-called good cholesterol. Having high HDL is associated with a lower risk of heart disease. Men should have an HDL level of greater than 40 mg/dl, and women, who naturally have a somewhat higher level of HDL, should have an HDL level of greater than 50 mg/dl.

Then there are triglycerides, the storage and transport form of fat. A triglyceride level of less than 150 mg/dl is normal. Finally, there is total cholesterol. That is a measured value that takes LDL, HDL, and triglycerides into consideration. Having a total cholesterol level of less than 200 mg/dl is associated with a lower risk of heart disease.

So what should you do if your cholesterol is outside the healthy range? The recommendations differ based on which type of cholesterol is abnormal.

**LDL and total cholesterol.** I lump these two together because elevated total cholesterol is often due to elevated LDL cholesterol. (On occasion, it's due to elevated HDL, and that is a good thing, so you don't need to do anything except keep up the good work.) The best way to bring down your LDL cholesterol is to eat a diet lower in saturated and trans fats and to lose weight.

Exercise will reduce also LDL cholesterol. Eating a diet lower in saturated and trans fats and exercising not only reduces the amount of LDL in your blood but it changes the characteristics of the LDL that's left behind. This new and improved LDL (large and fluffy instead of the evil small and dense LDL) remaining is much less likely to cause heart disease.

Bottom line: If your LDL is too high, cut the amount of saturated and trans fats in your diet and add exercise.

**HDL cholesterol.** Since this is the good cholesterol, in general, the more HDL you have, the better off you are. Increasing the amount of good fat in your diet will increase HDL. By good fat, I mean, of course, not the fat from meats but that from plants and seeds and seafood. Polyunsaturated fats, corn oil, for example, as well as monounsaturated fats (olive oil or canola oil) will bring up HDL. The omega fatty acids found in seafood will, too.

Eating saturated fats from meat will increase your HDL but will increase your LDL as well, so they cancel each other out. Exercise will also help increase your good cholesterol. Current research suggests that this occurs primarily by reducing insulin resistance. (For more information on insulin resistance, check out the section on metabolic syndrome on page 317.)

Modest consumption of alcohol will elevate your HDL. It's not a reason to take up drinking, but it is one more reason to enjoy the occasional glass of wine if you already drink.

Estrogen increases HDL levels; that's why women have a higher baseline HDL than men, at least before menopause. And it was one of the reasons that hormone therapy after menopause was advocated in the last century, but it didn't work. Researchers found that women on hormone therapy who were taking estrogen plus progesterone had a slightly higher rate of heart disease than women who didn't. Health food stores are trying to promote eating natural estrogens found in plants—they're called phytoestrogens—using the argument that these foods or drugs will increase HDL levels. They may, but it's clear that the relationship between estrogen and heart disease isn't a straightforward "more-is-less" type of deal. More research is needed on this topic before phytoestrogens can be medically recommended.

Bottom line: A diet rich in good fats and low in bad fats is the best way to increase your HDL. Alcohol and exercise will also help.

**Triglycerides.** Finally, let's talk about triglycerides. These are maybe the most interesting part of the whole lipid profile and have only gotten attention very recently. Triglycerides are the storage form of fats in your body. Plain fat is hydrophobic and doesn't mix well with water. In triglycerides, fats are linked to a carbohydrate backbone, and that allows them to deal with the watery world of our bodies. Fat deposits throughout the body are basically stockpiles of triglycerides. Mostly, those stay put. There are triglycerides in the blood as well. These are fats on their way somewhere—either to be used by the cells or stored in fat deposits.

Here's what's interesting about triglycerides: For many people, the amount of triglycerides in the blood is due not to how much fat was in the most recent meal, but how much carbohydrate. Triglyceride levels increase after a meal high in carbohydrates. Pretty amazing. Although the exact physiology of this phenomenon hasn't been completely worked out, it looks as though the people most likely to have this tendency are those with insulin resistance.

Given the link between triglycerides, insulin resistance, and heart disease, it is important to eat a diet relatively high in good fats and to make the carbohydrates that you eat whole grains, nuts, and other foods with a low glycemic load. Those of you with high triglycerides should replace potatoes and starches in your diet with nuts, olive oil, and seafood, which contain good fats, and fruits, vegetables, and whole grains (brown breads rather than white bread; old-fashioned oatmeal over instant; beans rather than pasta) to maximally reduce your triglycerides.

## DIABETES

This disease increases the risk of heart disease dramatically, because having elevated glucose levels damages the blood vessels and makes it easier for people with diabetes to develop narrowed arteries in the heart and throughout the body. Because of this increased risk of heart disease, it is essential that other risk factors like high blood pressure, high cholesterol, and smoking be well managed.

How people with diabetes should eat has been the source of much controversy over the past few decades. Initially, it was thought that they should avoid sweets and sugar. As understanding of carbohydrate metabolism grew, and it was understood that all carbohydrates turn to sugar in the body, all carbohydrates were declared equal, and the move was toward spreading them throughout the day to achieve predictable and controllable blood sugar levels, even in the hour or so after eating a meal.

Until recently, people with diabetes were almost universally put on low-fat, high-carbohydrate diets because of concerns about the elevated cardiac risk they faced. Now there is some movement away from the low-fat diet to one that allows more fat and fewer carbohydrates.

The carbohydrates eaten by diabetics should have a low glycemic load. This means choosing fruits, vegetables, and whole grains over starches, breads, and refined foods. People with diabetes should not necessarily decrease the total amount of fat in their diets but should chose more mono- and polyunsaturated fats and omega fats instead of saturated fat. In practice this means more lean meat and fish, more nuts and olive oil. And fewer starches—less pasta, less rice, and fewer potatoes, but more vegetables. If this sounds a lot like the advice given to those with low HDL and those with high triglycerides, it is. And that's because all three problems—diabetes, low HDL, and high triglycerides—are caused by the same underlying factor: insulin resistance. So you shouldn't be surprised that the treatment is the same.

Weight loss will improve insulin resistance. A brisk 30-minute walk 5 to 7 days a week will help keep your sugars in line. Losing 10 percent of your weight will improve your blood pressure, lower your cholesterol, and improve your glycemic control.

Daily goals for sugar should be a morning fasting glucose of 80 to 120 mg/dl and glucose between 100 and 140 mg/dl before going to bed at night. Long-term control of glucose is adequate when your measured hemoglobin A1c—that's the measure of long-term glucose control—is less than 6.5 percent.

## HIGH BLOOD PRESSURE

Until very recently, a normal blood pressure was one that was less than 140/90 millimeters of mercury (mm Hg). Recommendations published in 2002 are that people with blood pressure between 120/80 to 140/90 be considered well on their way to high blood pressure and be counseled to lose weight, exercise, and eat a low-salt diet to try to reduce their risk of moving into the frankly hypertensive category. This means millions more people will have "abnormal" blood pressure and as such are at increased risk of heart disease.

For people with diabetes or serious kidney disease, normal blood pressure should not exceed 125/80. Elevated blood pressure can increase risk of stroke, heart disease, and kidney disease.

Doctors could measure blood pressure and had known its risks long before we had any medicines for treating it. At that point, diet and lifestyle change were really the only tools we had to combat this deadly disease. (Sound familiar?)

The tendency to develop high blood pressure is inherited. If one or both of your parents had high blood pressure, you are at pretty high risk of developing it as well. Even so, biology is not destiny. So what lowers blood pressure? Just about everything that's good for you: exercising daily, reducing your weight, eating more fruits and vegetables, and finally, eating less salt (sodium) will all help you reduce your blood pressure.

As difficult as all those changes may be, lowering sodium intake may be the toughest. Sodium is added to almost all processed foods. It's one of the oldest and still most widely used forms of preserving food. I frequently challenge my students to try to lower their salt intake just so they'll appreciate firsthand how tough this is. Sodium is everywhere. The salt you put on your food is just a drop in the bucket of the sodium that makes its way into your body every day. Given that, how can you moderate your sodium intake?

Salt is an important preservative and a convenient way for manufacturers to add flavor to processed foods. So virtually everything that is processed is loaded with sodium. If they take the salt out, the food doesn't taste like anything at all. So, here's the most important tip in how to follow a low-sodium diet: Avoid prepared foods. This includes prepared meals that are frozen or that come in cans. Spaghetti topped with tomato sauce that you cook at home with fresh tomatoes can contain just a few milligrams of sodium. Chef

Boyardee canned spaghetti has 1,100 milligrams of sodium. Even Healthy Choice frozen spaghetti dinner has almost 500 milligrams of sodium per serving.

What's the right amount of sodium in a low-sodium diet? The recommended amount of salt (sodium chloride) for those with high blood pressure is 580 milligrams per day. The only way to get there is to eat primarily fresh foods and have the only salt in the food be what you add for flavor.

It's a challenge. And a very tough goal when so many of us depend on prepackaged foods at home and eat out frequently. Nevertheless, studies have shown that sticking to a low-sodium diet brings blood pressure down by as much as 11 mm Hg. For many people, this makes the difference between having to take high blood pressure medication or not. Try it. The amount of sodium in every food is listed on the nutrition label. Keep track of where your sodium comes from and see if you can bring it down.

So here's how to follow a low-sodium diet.

1. Avoid prepared foods.
2. Avoid foods that are: canned, cured (like bacon), pickled (in brine), or smoked (ham).
3. Avoid condiments such as MSG (monosodium glutamate), ketchup, mustard, and soy sauce.
4. Don't add salt to the cooking water for vegetables, rice, or pasta.
5. Rinse canned foods to remove some of the sodium.
6. Buy low-sodium canned or prepackaged foods.

Bottom line: If you have high blood pressure, eat a diet rich in fruits and vegetables and low in sodium, and exercise as often as you can. Eat fresh whenever possible.

# HEART DISEASE

Once you have had a heart attack or angina or an angioplasty, your cardiologist will very likely encourage you to see a nutritionist to help you change the way you eat. The nutritionist will probably want you to go on a low-fat, high-carbohydrate diet. A fat-counting diet, which dramatically limits saturated fats, has been shown to reverse heart disease.

Is a low-fat high-carb the best diet for those with heart disease? Not necessarily. Any diet that restricts saturated fat and cholesterol and emphasizes fresh vegetables, whole grains, and fish will lower your risk of having a second heart attack. The Mediterranean diet, as it has come to be known, fits this bill. Based on the Seven Countries study done in seven Mediterranean countries associated with a lower risk of heart disease, this diet emphasizes fresh fruits and vegetables, olive oil and other monounsaturated fats, fish and chicken over beef, whole grains over processed flours, and moderate consumption of wine.

A four-year study compared this diet to the low-fat diet normally recommended and found that the Mediterranean diet was associated with a 50 percent reduction in risk of a second heart attack. So, even after a heart attack, there is choice about how to change your diet to improve your health, while still finding one you can enjoy and stick to. Here are some tips on how to eat if you have heart disease.

1. Incorporate nuts into your daily eating plan. These are a great source of protein and good fats.

2. Make sure the carbohydrates you eat are low-glycemic-load foods. Aim for foods with a glycemic load of less than 20. This means more fruits and vegetables, whole-grain breads and crackers, with few pastries, cookies, and breads made from refined flour.

3. Many low-fat meals center on a starchy carbohydrate; these foods tend to have a higher glycemic load than fruits and vegetables. Because of this, you should reduce the amount of starchy carbohydrates (like rice, noodles, or pasta) and increase the amount of fruits and vegetables. Cutting the starch in half and doubling the other carbohydrates will help you control your insulin levels.

4. Make most of the meat that you eat fish and other seafood.

5. When you do eat meat, make sure you choose the leanest meats, with more poultry than pork, more pork than beef.

6. When you eat dairy products, make sure you are eating the low-fat version.

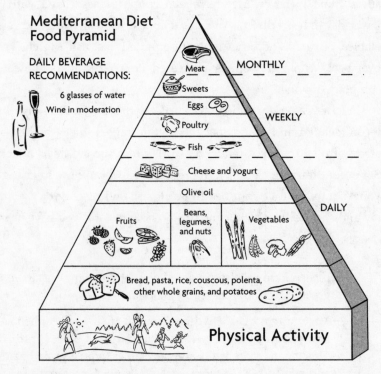

## Mediterranean Diet Food Pyramid

**DAILY BEVERAGE RECOMMENDATIONS:**

6 glasses of water
Wine in moderation

Meat — MONTHLY
Sweets
Eggs
Poultry — WEEKLY
Fish
Cheese and yogurt
Olive oil
Fruits — Beans, legumes, and nuts — Vegetables — DAILY
Bread, pasta, rice, couscous, polenta, other whole grains, and potatoes

**Physical Activity**

© 2000 Oldways Preservation & Exchange Trust          www.oldwayspt.org

7. Avoid trans fats. Check food labels for the presence of partially hydrogenated oils, and if it has them, put it back on the shelf.

8. Watch your calories.

## METABOLIC SYNDROME

If you scored 3 points or higher on the section about metabolic syndrome, then you have it—but you shouldn't feel alone. Based on this definition, almost one-quarter of all Americans do.

So what is metabolic syndrome? It is a group of abnormalities that tend to run together and dramatically increase an individual's risk of heart disease. This phenomenon was first described in 1988 by Gerald Reaven, M.D., an endocrinologist at Stanford University who noticed that many of his patients who had high blood pressure also had diabetes, or at least a higher-than-normal blood glucose level. Also, many of them had trunkal obesity, that is, they carried their excess weight predominately around their waists. Plus, many of them also had abnormal cholesterol with elevated triglyceride levels and low levels of HDL.

All of these problems were linked by a single cause: Their bodies were resistant to the effects of what is probably the most complex and important hormone in our bodies: insulin. Most people have heard about insulin because some people with diabetes don't have enough of it and must give themselves insulin injections in order to live. That's because one of insulin's most important jobs (though not by any means its only job) is to help cells take up glucose from the bloodstream. People who have insulin resistance need much higher levels of insulin to get that job done. When your body can't produce enough insulin to meet your ever increasing demand, you have diabetes.

You know that once you develop diabetes your risk of heart disease increases dramatically. But did you know that just being insulin resistant and having high levels of insulin in your body day after day also increases your risk of heart disease? That's because insulin has many jobs in the body, and having higher than normal levels of insulin changes the way insulin goes about doing some of these other jobs.

For example, high levels of insulin cause the body to hold on to salt, which in turn makes the body hold on to water, which can cause high blood pressure. High insulin also encourages fat to accumulate around your waist. Abdominal fat is the most metabolically active fat; that means that it is the easiest to put on and the easiest to take off. So if you lose weight, you will probably lose at least some of that fat. That's the good news. The bad news is that abdominal fat is associated with higher rates of cardiac disease. High insulin levels also help turn carbohydrates into fats.

All this adds up to a higher risk of heart disease. How much higher? It looks as if it could increase your odds of having heart disease by as much as 400 percent. If you are under 35 and a woman, your risk of having a heart attack is very low, so an increase of 400 percent, while it sounds scary, probably doesn't increase your real risk of a heart attack very much. But if you are a woman approaching menopause or a man, then your baseline risk is greater, and a 400 percent increase can really make a difference.

The tendency to develop insulin resistance is inherited. But, it's not like having blue eyes, where you either have it or you don't. It's the *tendency* to develop insulin resistance, like the tendency to be a good athlete. The possibility is there, but you have to do certain things for it to develop. It's nature plus nurture.

So what can nurture this trait? Obesity can. Not everyone with insulin resistance is overweight, but if you are overweight and have this inborn predisposition, it will bring it out.

Having a sedentary lifestyle will, too. Muscles play an important role in taking glucose up out of the blood. If they are not being used, they don't take up as much glucose, and somehow that sets the stage for insulin resistance.

If there are factors that promote the development of insulin resistance and metabolic syndrome, are there factors that reduce the likelihood of developing it? There are. Exercise is the most powerful factor, and it's surprising how little you need for therapeutic effect. A brisk daily walk lasting half an hour will reduce the likelihood of developing insulin resistance by almost 50 percent.

What you eat also makes a difference in whether or not you develop insulin resistance. A diet rich in whole grains and fruits and vegetables and low in sugary drinks is associated with a lower risk. A high-fiber diet is also associated with a lower risk of developing metabolic syndrome. And, finally, and perhaps most surprisingly, a diet rich in dairy products is associated with a much lower risk of developing metabolic syndrome.

Of course, if you are reading this, chances are you already have metabolic syndrome. So now what? In general, the same things that reduce your chance of developing metabolic syndrome will also help you get rid of it by reducing your level of insulin resistance.

So, weight loss will certainly reverse much of the insulin resistance you have developed. That's just one more reason to keep trying to achieve the proper weight. But until then, eating a diet that is high in fiber, high in low-fat dairy products, and high in whole grains and vegetables will help. Exercise also is extremely helpful.

One last thing: If you have metabolic syndrome with high triglycerides, then you should probably avoid the low-fat, high-carbohydrate diet. Individuals with insulin resistance have this amazing ability to turn carbohydrates into fats. Dr. Reaven, the endocrinologist who first described metabolic syndrome, recommends a diet high in monounsaturated fats (like those in olive oil, canola oil, and nuts) and relatively low in carbohydrates.

Dr. Reaven's perfect diet would include 40 percent of daily calories from monounsaturated fats and about the same from carbohydrates. Moreover, the carbs that you do eat should be fruits and vegetables or whole grains. Refined carbohydrates should be avoided.

They turn rapidly into glucose once you eat them and promote the release of high levels of insulin, and that only makes the whole business worse.

Bottom line: If you have metabolic syndrome, you should follow these guidelines:

1. Eat a diet high in monounsaturated fats. (For more information on what kinds of foods are high in monounsaturated fats, see "Know Your Fats," page 240.)

2. Eat fruits and vegetables daily.

3. Avoid refined carbohydrates.

4. Eat a diet rich in low-fat or reduced-fat dairy products.

5. Try to take a brisk walk or get 30 minutes of exercise every day.

## FAMILY MEDICAL HISTORY

If your parents had heart disease at an early age, or any of the associated risk factors of heart disease—diabetes, high blood pressure, or high cholesterol—then you are at risk of developing these diseases as well.

A heart attack before the age of 45 in a man or 55 in a woman is an unusual event, though not nearly unusual enough. If your mother or father had one, then that increases the chance that you will develop heart disease as well. How much that risk is increased isn't known, but a family history of heart disease at an early age is a signal to doctors—and should be to patients—that risk factors should be screened for and well controlled to reduce that risk as much as possible.

If one of your parents had diabetes, then you are also at risk of developing diabetes. Fortunately, being at risk doesn't mean you will—it means you could. A study published in *The New England*

*Journal of Medicine* in 2002 showed that even people at very high risk of developing diabetes—those with insulin resistance—could prevent that by losing some weight and exercising. The participants in this study lost 7 percent of their initial body weight over the course of 6 months and kept most of that off. Losing that much weight prevented most of them from developing diabetes. People in the study were asked to engage in moderate exercise (they sweat lightly but were still able to talk) for 150 minutes a week, just over 20 minutes a day.

If you have a family history of diabetes, you can dramatically reduce your risk of developing diabetes as well by maintaining a healthy weight and exercising daily. When I talk about diabetes, I am talking about what is called adult onset diabetes, or type 2 diabetes, which can be treated with pills as well as insulin. The other type of diabetes—juvenile, or type 1, diabetes—must always be treated with insulin, and does not run in families.

What about high blood pressure? All of us are at risk of developing high blood pressure eventually. Half of everyone over the age of 60 has it. If either of your parents have high blood pressure, then you too are at a higher risk of developing it as well. What can you do to reduce or prevent it? The answers are probably what you would expect.

1. Lose weight. In one study an average weight loss of just 8 pounds cut the risk of developing high blood pressure in half.

2. Reduce salt intake. Researchers found that cutting salt to less than 6 grams per day dropped blood pressure by an average of 3 mm Hg. That may not sound like much to you, but in the Framingham population studies, a 2 mm Hg drop in blood pressure reduced the risk of developing high blood pressure by 20 percent.

3. Exercise. Moderate exercise done 30 minutes per day, most days of the week, will reduce blood pressure by 4 mm Hg.

4. Reduce your alcohol intake. A number of studies have shown that reducing alcohol intake to no more than two drinks per day for men and one drink per day for women lowered blood pressure by 4 mm Hg.

5. Eat a diet high in potassium. Eating bananas, oranges, or leafy greens daily was associated with a 2 mm Hg drop in blood pressure.

6. Eat a diet rich in fruits, fresh vegetables, and low-fat dairy products and low in saturated fats. This diet was associated with a 4mm Hg drop in blood pressure.

Finally, what about cholesterol? If you have a family history of high cholesterol, then you may be at risk for high cholesterol yourself. Obviously, diet is a major contributor in the development of high cholesterol, but your genes speak here as well. The newest recommendations from the National Institutes of Health are that everyone over the age of 20 should have their cholesterol measured every five years.

This is a much younger age at which to start screening than had been previously recommended, so if you are under the age of 40, you may not have had your cholesterol checked. You should discuss this with your doctor and see if she wants to measure it now.

Certainly if you have a family history of high cholesterol or early heart disease or if you have diabetes, you should seriously consider having your cholesterol checked at regular intervals. Your risk of developing high cholesterol if you have a family history of it isn't clear at this point. But even if you don't have high cholesterol now, you should certainly consider eating a diet low in saturated fat. Diet alone can bring down cholesterol 10 to 15 percent on average, and that may be all you really need at this point. For more information on how to eat a low-saturated-fat diet, see chapter 9.

# CHAPTER 12
## FAMILY HERITAGE

### YOUR FAMILY INHERITANCE: NATURE

If you scored 5 or more in the section titled How You Are Shaped by Nature there is a good chance that you have inherited traits from your family that affect your ability to control your weight. It's easy to imagine that a tendency to gain weight is as inherited as having red hair or being tall or having broad shoulders. Recent studies have put a finer point on it: Genes govern not only where you put on weight but also how you get fat. That is to say, it's not just the body that gets handed down to you, but the behavior you'll likely use to run it as well.

Most of us observe something among our friends when we're young. If the parents of a family are overweight, then the kids are more likely to be overweight, too. It used to be thought that this was due to the shared environment: You were taught about food and how to eat by your parents. If they overate, they would teach you to overeat as well. The environment does play a powerful role, but research done within the past two decades suggests that there is also a strong genetic component.

Albert Stunkard, M.D., one of the pioneers in the science of obesity, asked this question: Is the tendency to gain weight inherited or learned? He then looked at children who were adopted and compared their weights to the weights of both their adopted and biological parents. He found that the adopted children were much more likely to have the same body-weight class as their biological parents rather than their adopted parents. It wasn't true in 100 percent of cases, but it was significant. Much more than would be expected if it were just a coincidence.

Then Dr. Stunkard asked another question: How big a role did genes play? In order to answer this question, he looked at obesity in identical and fraternal twins. Identical twins share the exact same genes. Fraternal twins share exactly half the same set of genes. (The same as any two siblings would.) Dr. Stunkard looked at twins who were raised together and compared them with twins raised separately. If some certain trait showed up more commonly among identical twins than in fraternal twins, then it would seem obvious that the trait was more likely due to their genes rather than their environment. That's the theory, and twin studies have been used extensively in figuring out what is nature, or inborn, and what is nurture, or learned.

In Europe it's easy to find twins. You simply contact—I'm not making this up—the Swedish Twins Registry. There are about 25,000 twins on file there, so Dr. Stunkard tracked down about 600 pairs of twins born between 1886 and 1958. Of these, about 100 were identical twins who were raised in the same home and 100 were identical twins raised apart. He also located 200 fraternal pairs raised together and 200 who were raised separately. Then he compared the body mass indexes (BMIs) of each twin pair.

He found that the twins who were raised together were more likely to have the same bodies. So environment does count. But he also found that fraternal twins raised apart were likely to share the same body shape. And here's what's most surprising: More than two-thirds of the identical twins who were raised apart had the same BMI.

So there is clearly a very important genetic component to weight gain. But how does a genetic predisposition express itself? One genetic trait is how well you burn off calories. Although there aren't big differences in basic metabolic rates, there is a difference in how active people are. And I'm not referring to whether you are an athlete or not, but to the activity of daily life. Whether you are a toe-tapping fidgeter or a serene Buddha is an inherited quality. And fidgeters burn off more calories than those who are able to sit still. It's not a lot of calories and certainly can't account for all of the weight.

So researchers started looking at eating behaviors and asked the question, are these behaviors inherited? Food preference was known to have some inherited quality—sensitivity to bitter foods has been well described (see page 284 for information about those who have this sensitivity), but its link to obesity was not clear. So once again researchers turned to twins to answer that question.

American researchers recruited 2,300 pairs of twins over the age of 50 (they had to advertise for them). Each of the twins filled out a questionnaire about what he or she ate. The researchers then divided the eaters into one of two broad categories: those who ate lots of veggies and whole grains (your basic healthy diet) and those who ate lots of fats and sweets (your basic all-American, unhealthy diet). And then they compared the twins to see how often they fell into the same pattern-of-eating category.

There was no pattern in the unhealthy dieters. Whether they were identical twins or fraternal twins didn't matter. And, curiously, none of the women seemed to show the effect of any genetic influence. But men who ate a healthy diet did show evidence of a genetic component: If one of the identical twin men had a healthy pattern of eating, there was a very good chance that his brother did, too. Fraternal twins had about half as much a chance as the identical twins. So there does appear to be a genetic component in food choice, especially the (now) unusual choice to eat a healthy diet.

What all this means is that, while there is a genetic component to food preference, it may not be powerful enough to overcome the cultural pressures to eat in a less healthy way.

There are other eating behaviors that seem to have a genetic component to them, like disinhibition, or the inability to put on the eating brakes when set off by some trigger—a food you really like or even seeing someone else overeat, for example. You'd think this behavior was learned, but it's not. Researchers followed a large Amish population in Pennsylvania, looking at this behavior. They chose the Amish because they are socially isolated and the family tree was well known back to the eighteenth century. Researchers interviewed hundreds of Amish people from sixty-five families whose kinship was well known, and tracing these families back, scientists found that disinhibition was much more likely to run in families than not.

Is biology destiny? Or as one of my patients put it, "Am I destined to be fat like my parents and sisters?" Obviously, the answer is no. Not every identical twin ended up the same; genetics is only one component of who we are and how we live.

On the other hand, life is not fair. I'm telling you about the role of genetics so that you'll understand that when it comes to gaining weight or losing it, we are not all playing on the same level field. Genes definitely make it harder for some people to gain weight or to lose it. That doesn't mean you should be defeatist or fatalistic about losing weight if the genetic deck seems stacked against you. It means you have to understand where you have an advantage or disadvantage, and take that into account when you're designing your weight-management program.

It's just harder for some people to lose weight than it is for others. You know it. I know it. And now doctors know it, too. That's why your diet and your lifestyle have to be tailored to fit you. One size doesn't fit all, because it doesn't take into consideration all the ways in which we are different. If you can figure out what works for you and you alone, the hardest part of your work will be done.

## YOUR FAMILY INHERITANCE: NURTURE

If you scored 25 points or more in the section called How You Are Shaped by Nurture, then your experiences with food and activity as a child may be contributing to your difficulties in managing your weight as an adult.

In this section, we look at your family's attitude toward food and exercise, because there is evidence that these attitudes, shaped early in life, can influence how you feel about food and exercise as an adult.

Let's talk about food first. The way food was made available in your childhood can have an impact on the way you view food as an adult. Kids up to the age of 3 are able to regulate how much food they eat based on internal cues of satiety. After that point, though, external cues become more important: cues like serving size and parental expectations.

Attitudes about food are developed early in life. Many of my patients report having food used as a reward for achievement or a treatment for psychic or physical ills, and for many of them these links have persisted into adulthood. After a long day at work, Janet feels that she "deserves" a big bowl of ice cream as a reward. And when she doesn't have it, she feels punished, deprived. It has been a struggle for her to address this sense that food is a reward. I hear this over and over again from my patients and my friends: Food is a reward, a comfort, therapy.

This sense of food is learned, of course, but on a biological level, food is literally a reward. Voltaire recognized this as early as the eighteenth century when he said, "Nothing would be more tiresome than eating and drinking if God had not made them a pleasure as well as a necessity." Eating and drinking are two of the most primal pleasures that we have—right up there with sex and sleeping.

But food, the easiest legitimate trigger in our culture to obtain and indulge, is not the only thing that tickles our pleasure centers. Many other activities do as well. Exercise is the most widely touted and probably the best. The various magazines devoted to these pursuits still print articles that describe all the hormonal changes that take place in the body when it exercises, the great feelings that surge after a workout, and the near-spiritual quality of the "endorphin high." Hobbies and other pursuits can also trigger our pleasure centers. Studies done on recreational activities, even though as ordinary as sewing or gardening, show that they can lower heart rates and blood pressure and tickle our endorphins. Meditation has many of the same effects as opiates, except that it doesn't interfere with our ability to drive, make us drool, or make us say things to our friends that provoke head-slapping remorse the next morning.

Our link between food and pleasure is obvious; it's reinforced biologically at least three times a day and often explicitly used as a reward from early childhood. The other pleasure triggers aren't as well established for us. Few of us were taught to meditate as children to help us cope with the injuries to body and soul. Not when there were cookies at hand. So, many of us are forced to try to decode and reprogram this link ourselves as adults. It can be done. It's just a little harder.

One of the ways we make the link between other activities and pleasure is by engaging in them as a family. Families who pursue pleasurable activities together, like sports or hiking or gardening or fishing, are teaching kids about other ways to get rewards. The only thing my family did together was to eat, and our Sunday dinners were without a doubt the best part of our week. But there were two activities my mother did with me and my sisters: She took us to the public library every Saturday, and she taught us how to sew. And to this day, both reading and sewing remain two of my favorite activities.

Exercise that starts early in life has a greater chance of remaining pleasurable and important to us as adults. Few things in life are better at predicting an active adulthood as participating in sports or other physical activities in childhood. But if you didn't learn a sport or hobby as a child, you aren't doomed; it's never too late. It's part of the baggage you brought from childhood, and it has to be unloaded. You are not just the child your parents wanted you to be. As an adult, you have made decisions about who you wanted to be and what you wanted to do that were based on your own needs, desires, and goals. The genetic and environmental baggage that you were saddled with as a kid does not determine who you are now.

Learn to recognize childhood habits that are ingrained in your attitudes about food and exercise. Then resolve to reshape those attitudes into ones that are more compatible with your adult goals— with who you are and what you want to do with your life and your body now.

Nature isn't destiny; nurture isn't destiny. They do have an impact on how hard your row is to hoe—to deny that would be to ignore what science tells us. But neither do they determine what can and can't be done. Only we can determine that.

# 13 CHAPTER

# EATING HABITS

I F YOU HAVE A score of 10 or more in the Eating Habits section of the questionnaire, chances are good that how you eat is contributing to your difficulty in losing weight or maintaining your weight. Welcome to the club. Science has only recently tried to figure out how the way that we eat affects our ability to maintain our ideal weight.

In this section of the questionnaire, I look at several aspects of your eating habits: skipping meals, snacking between meals, and hunger. As you can see, these are very different (albeit related) topics, and it's not hard to imagine that they may affect whether you gain or lose weight, although how they do that may surprise you.

Later in the chapter, we'll look at the roles played by emotions and habit in eating.

## SKIPPING MEALS

When I ask patients how they are trying to lose weight, I find that a common strategy is to skip meals or to eat only one meal per day. You know what? It doesn't work. Many of my patients tell me that they don't eat breakfast. By skipping breakfast they figure they will be able to consume fewer calories during the day, because they will be eating only two meals rather than three. That's the theory.

Here's the reality: In multiple studies done in a variety of populations, people who eat breakfast are much less likely to be overweight than people who don't.

Some of my patients tell me that they are not hungry at breakfast time, and that may well be true. There are aspects of meal scheduling and hunger that are learned; that's why we are hungry every 4 to 5 hours during the day but can go for 8 hours overnight as we sleep. If you are out of the habit of breakfast, you will not get hungry for it. Once you start, however, you will find yourself anticipating the meal and getting hungry for it as you do for your other meals.

The other comment I hear from some people is that they get hungry just a couple of hours after eating breakfast and feel as though they stay hungry for the rest of the morning. This is, I think, more a function of what they eat for breakfast than the fact that they are eating breakfast. The most common type of adult breakfast is a quick donut, muffin, roll, or toast and coffee. This breakfast may, in fact, make you hungry just a couple of hours later, because it's not very much to eat, and it doesn't stick around very long.

Foods containing only refined flour and maybe some fat contain a lot of calories but aren't very satiating. If you ate a plain bagel with cream cheese, you would be eating just over 600 calories. A blueberry muffin with raisins and a smear of butter—that's almost 500 calories.

A couple of donuts from Dunkin' Donuts will run you 580 calories. Add a cup o' joe with some milk, and you have what is currently the great American breakfast. According to my patients (as well as my own extensive personal experience), a couple of hours after this kind of breakfast, you find yourself at the snack machine eyeing a bag of cheese puffs, just a little something to tide you over until lunchtime.

So, what should you eat for breakfast? Well, in a survey of 122 healthy older men and women in Madrid, Spain, those who were a normal weight ate a more varied breakfast, eating from both a greater number of foods and more groups of foods. They also spent a longer time eating their breakfasts and consumed greater quantities of food than did their overweight counterparts.

So eating a variety of foods and eating enough food is good. A more specific recommendation depends on your diet and the foods you like. In general, I tend to recommend either a high-fiber cereal with fruit and maybe a piece of toast with peanut butter or, if you are counting carbohydrates, something that provides protein with a minimal amount of saturated fat—maybe a poached egg with a couple of slices of Canadian bacon. Just compare the calories.

| | |
|---|---|
| ½ cup All-Bran with fat-free milk | 120 calories |
| 1 slice of toast with 1 teaspoon peanut butter | 135 calories |
| ½ cantaloupe | 100 calories |
| Total | 355 calories |

How about an omelet?

| | |
|---|---|
| Omelet made with 2 whole eggs and 1 egg white | 185 calories |
| 1 ounce cheese, added to the omelet | 115 calories |
| 2 slices of Canadian bacon | 90 calories |
| Total | 390 calories |

These breakfasts stand a much better chance of getting you to lunchtime without the trip to the snack machine. You don't have to take my word for it. At the VA Medical Center in Minneapolis, four-teen men were served either a low-fiber cereal or a high-fiber cereal in the morning. Four hours later they were offered lunch—all they could eat. Each subject filled out a questionnaire before the lunch asking them how hungry they were. Those who ate the high-fiber ce-real were less hungry, and they also ate less at lunch than did their low-fiber-cereal counterparts. The fiber sticks with you; you feel full for longer. So you may not need the snack machine, and you might even eat less at lunch.

There is no similar study for a low-carbohydrate version of this breakfast, comparing say, donuts with the omelet-and-bacon break-fast. In studies, subjects on the low-carb diet ate fewer calories per day than their counterparts on other diets without experiencing ex-cess hunger. The high satiating qualities of proteins is one of the most effective aspects of a low-carb diet.

Eating breakfast even makes you smarter! In several studies published over the past 25 years, when individuals who have had breakfast are given tasks that require concentration and memory, they do better than their unbreakfasted counterparts.

So maybe eating breakfast makes you smarter, and maybe more thin people eat breakfast, but does it help you get thinner and stay thinner? There is research that suggests it does. At Vanderbilt Uni-versity, fifty-two women were divided into two groups and put on a 12-week diet. Both were supposed to eat the same number of calories per day, but one group was supposed to eat breakfast and the other was supposed to skip breakfast. Everybody lost weight—an average of 17 pounds in 12 weeks—but those who ate breakfast reported less hunger and less impulsive snacking.

And successful dieters are much more likely to eat breakfast than the average American. The National Weight Control Registry, a group of three thousand men and women who are successful dieters (on average they have lost more than 60 pounds and kept it off for more than 6 years) were surveyed about their eating habits, and almost 80 percent said they ate breakfast every day. Only 4 percent reported that they never ate breakfast. Statistics on adult eating habits are hard to come by, but in a recent Gallup poll on children, fewer than half said that they ate breakfast. I can only imagine that the rate among adults is even lower.

One last word on breakfast: Sumo wrestlers skip breakfast. It's part of their centuries-old tradition of gaining weight. It works for them, and trust me, it can work for you, too. So, eat breakfast, but make it worth your while by eating a variety of low-fat, high-fiber foods.

What about skipping other meals? One of the problems when you skip a meal is that you get hungry, and when you get hungry, it is very hard to stop eating when you've had enough. One of the primary predictors of how much someone is going to eat at a given time is how hungry they are when they sit down at the table. If you eat only one meal a day, you give up control of your eating when you finally sit down for that meal, because you're starved.

And being that hungry makes overeating easy. You haven't eaten all day, and the hungrier you are, the faster you tend to eat. You shovel it in, and the mechanisms that are in place to tell you to stop are overwhelmed. By the time your body tells you that you have eaten enough, you have eaten way more than enough.

There is also evidence that being without food causes the stress hormones in your body to get revved up. You don't even have to go all day without eating to get your stress hormones going. In a study published in *The New England Journal of Medicine*, researchers looked at the effect of two types of eating: nibbling and gorging. Men assigned to the nibbling group ate seventeen snacks over the course of the day but no big meals. Gorgers ate the more traditional three meals per day. The researchers were mostly interested in seeing if changing how these men ate would change their cholesterol, but they measured other body chemicals as well. Nibbling definitely improved the men's cholesterol, but in addition, the researchers found that the nibblers had much lower levels of the hormone associated with stress.

Not eating is a stress on the body, so it's not really surprising that being hungry would cause a higher level of stress hormone. This is a problem when you are trying to lose weight, because stress makes you fat. The hormones your body puts out when you are stressed, either because of events in your life or because you haven't eaten, direct your body to stop burning fat. And chronic stress makes you put the fat on in a particular area—your stomach. So by skipping meals, you are actually making yourself fatter, not thinner.

The other problem with eating only one meal per day is that one meal isn't really enough. What happens then is snacking. With many people who eat only one meal per day, that one meal lasts all evening long.

So, how many meals is the right amount—three, five, seventeen? There is some evidence that how many meals is not as important as the day-to-day pattern of eating. Overeating occurs more frequently in those who don't have a regular pattern. A number of analyses indicate that whether you eat three, five, or ten meals or snacks has little direct effect on energy balance. It's not the actual number of meals that is most important, but it's consistency on a daily basis.

In a recent study, researchers found that high day-to-day variation in energy intakes were associated with higher fat and BMI. A degree of regularity and structure to daily eating may also reduce the chances for opportunistic or emotion-driven breakdowns in dietary restraint.

Bottom line: Eat breakfast every day, and try to maintain a pattern of eating that keeps you from getting hungry and that you can stick with routinely.

## SNACKING AND HUNGER

So is there anything wrong with snacking if you get hungry between meals? No, it is important to eat when you are hungry and not let yourself get too hungry. On the other hand, there has been a pretty dramatic increase in the amount of food we consume as snacks versus meals, and this has paralleled our increasing weight as a nation. Over the past 25 years, our snacking has increased 200 percent—that is, the number of calories we take in as snacks—but our intake at mealtime has decreased only a very small amount. In other words, we are eating more snacks in addition to what we already eat.

Snacking can be helpful in weight control by keeping you from getting too hungry between meals. If you get too hungry, you end up eating much more at a meal than you otherwise might. Also, when you are hungry, your ability to avoid food that is appealing but not what you should eat diminishes dramatically.

When you find yourself snacking, ask yourself a few questions: First, why are you hungry now? One of the reasons that people get hungry is that the food they ate for their last meal didn't hold them until their next meal. If you have a couple of donuts for breakfast, it dramatically increases the chances that you will need a snack before lunch. In a study of fourteen men and women who were fed meals containing either high or low fiber content, hunger and the sensation of fullness lasted much, much longer after eating the meals with lots of fiber. Studies on other highly sating foods such as proteins have shown similar results. The meals you eat should contain foods that have high satiating powers to increase the chances that you will only get hungry in time for your next meal. So, the first thing you should question when you find yourself hungry between meals is why breakfast or lunch isn't holding.

Of course, it may not be what you ate for your last meal. Another common reason for getting hungry between meals is that the meal is delayed longer than earlier food can expect to hold you over. If you eat lunch at noon but dinner at 8:00 or 9:00 P.M., chances are you are going to get hungry before dinnertime.

Some people prefer to eat more frequently than the traditional three square meals per day. The three-meal eating pattern was forced on us by the demands of the industrial age, which allowed only one break during the workday to maximize productivity. So there is really no reason to consider three meals the magic number. You may be someone who prefers to eat more frequently.

If you like eating more frequently, that's fine, but, of course, you need to plan for this. Chances are that there is nothing in a snack machine that is good for you to eat. In general, the ideal snack should have some carbohydrate component to fill you up and some protein component to make it last. An apple with a small chunk of cheese is one obvious snack, a small container of yogurt is another. A handful of nuts is a good snack for those of you who are trying to limit carbohydrate intake. Probably none of these (except maybe the nuts) are going to be available at your local vending machine. So, if you are a snacker, take a snack with you to work or wherever you go. If you leave your snacking choices to the marketplace, you will end up taking in much more food than you need, and that will simply increase your food intake for the day. Who needs that?

This assumes that the reason you are snacking is because you are hungry. That's not always the case. People often snack for other reasons. Maybe you are bored or stressed. Or, and this is very common, maybe you have come to expect to snack when you engage in a particular activity—like watching television—and so the trigger to eat isn't hunger but something else.

When you find yourself cruising for a snack, first ask yourself, Am I hungry, or is this something else? When you are hungry, figure out why, and then go get yourself a snack you can work consistently into your everyday routine. If you are not hungry, figure out what the trigger is, and try to find some other activity to satisfy your need. I know: It's not easy! When you are stressed or upset, you may not even want to think about the big picture, but it's important.

You have to remember that your eating patterns are with you until you change them. They will not change on their own. If stress is an obvious trigger for you, then you have to deal with it more creatively. Once you do that, you have a much better chance of making a lasting change in the way you eat, even after you're at your ideal level.

Bottom line: Between-meal hunger may be due to meals of poorly satiating foods. Other possibilities include "hunger" due to emotional causes or a preference for more frequent meals. Make sure you eat meals that will last, and if you still want snacks, take them with you.

## EMOTIONAL EATING

If you scored 15 or more on the Emotional Eating section of the questionnaire, you have a tendency to eat out of habit rather than hunger. Or maybe you're using food to feed your spirit rather than your stomach. Both problems can add quite a few pounds. While the behaviors are the same—eating when you are not hungry—this section covers two very different phenomena: emotional eating and habitual eating. Let's start with emotional eating, then we'll talk about what I call mindless or habitual eating.

Feelings can make people eat. I'm not talking about feeling hunger, I'm talking about other kinds of feelings—emotions. Many of us eat in response to feelings—often bad feelings.

Judy, a 35-year-old divorced mother of two, finds herself in her office kitchen eating cookies whenever she gets angry or annoyed at a coworker. Just the act of putting that cookie in her mouth, she says, helps her get her thoughts together and figure out how to deal with her anger.

Janet, a 32-year-old legal assistant to a high-powered Washington, D.C., lawyer, rewards herself with a chunk of dark chocolate after a stressful day at the office. She feels like she "deserves" it.

Kathy, an energetic 42-year-old social worker and divorced mother of two teenage boys, comforts herself late at night with a big bowl of ice cream when her loneliness feels unbearable. She takes care of her clients, her family, and her friends, but at the end of the day she feels too drained to take care of herself. That's when the ice cream really helps.

Matt, a successful 40-year-old realtor, craves Skittles before going to make a million-dollar deal. Chewing these fruity bits on the way to the meeting gives him an outlet for the excitement he feels when "going in for the kill."

All of these people came to me for help in finding a diet that would allow them to take charge of their weight. Turning to food when confronted with overwhelming emotion seems as natural and inevitable to them—and to many of us—as scratching an itch or yawning with fatigue.

In order to understand that link, and ultimately break it, we have to understand the nature of stress and our bodies. In each instance, the desire for food comes in the face of overwhelming stress. It is a natural response—one programmed into us at a very primitive level, but one that leads to overeating, weight gain, and ultimately unhappiness.

Let's talk about stress—what it is and what it does to us. Our bodies' reaction to stress is something we share with most, if not all, species in the animal kingdom. We perceive a threat to our well-being—a big, hungry animal or a mugger—and immediately our bodies change in order to respond to that threat: Our hearts start to beat faster, we breathe faster, our eyes dilate, we stop digesting our food so that the blood that had been going to the gastrointestinal tract can go to our muscles. Thinking is slower, but reflex or gut responses are quicker. At the chemical level, we get a rush of adrenaline as well as another type of stress-response hormone: cortisol. All of these changes, known in sixth-grade biology terms as the fight-or-flight response, put us in peak form to cope with this life-threatening event.

That response worked great on the African savannah; in fact, without it we most certainly wouldn't have survived. But here in modern civilization it's not quite as useful. Sure, it's still helpful when the stressful event is something that requires either fight or flight—like a mugger in a dark alley—but most of our most stressful events in modern life are not direct threats to life and limb.

Modern life attacks us with emotional threats and stressors. But just because our physical being isn't threatened doesn't mean those stressors aren't important or painful. We all go through major life stresses that don't lay a hand on us: the death of someone we love, divorce, getting fired. And there are other stressors that affect us on a more regular basis: missing a plane, having a fight, disappointing someone, meeting deadlines. In many people these daily stresses also trigger that same life-or-death reaction: Adrenaline and cortisol start flowing; blood pressure, heart rate, and respiratory rate go up; and we're physically ready to fight off the attackers. Not very helpful in dealing with these kinds of stressors. And it's that response you are fighting when you tell yourself (on your good days, anyway), "Okay, take a deep breath. Calm down and deal."

Fight-or-flight is not well suited to the stresses we meet in our everyday lives. And chronic exposure to the stress response can make us fat and unhealthy. Over the past 20 years, researchers around the world have been interested in the effects of stress on health. In multiple studies, it has been shown that excessive and sustained cortisol are associated with depression, high blood pressure, osteoporosis, a suppressed immune system, and metabolic syndrome, along with higher rates of atherosclerosis and heart disease.

The physiology of this is still being worked out, but here's what we know so far: Adrenaline is the chemical that gets our hearts and lungs going and sends our blood pressure up. Cortisol has the job of finding the fuel to keep things running. Cortisol calls up the glucose we have stored in our livers and sends it to our brains, our hearts, our lungs, and our muscles to help us fight off an attacker or take off running. After the initial response to the stress is over, the adrenaline recedes, but the cortisol stays on to try to get things back to normal.

One of the things that cortisol does is to get us to eat; that way we can replace the glucose and fat that was liberated. Again, it worked well on the savannahs, but in response to deadlines and daily stress, we don't actually use that much of the freed fuel; most of it just ends up back in storage. Unfortunately, cortisol doesn't know that. It just goes about its job to get us to eat and we do, willingly. (The physiology of this is beautifully described in *Fight Fat After 40*, by Pamela Peeke, M.D., one of the scientists involved in this groundbreaking research. If you want to know more about how stress affects us, I highly recommend this book.)

We have already seen that, under stress, people head for sweets and fats and consume extra calories. It's not just humans who eat this way under stress. In a series of experiments, rats who were stressed by having a researcher pinch their tails were noted to eat even when they had just finished a meal and were probably not hungry. And when they ate, they preferred sweet and fatty rat food over their normal food.

There may be a biological reason for this preference for high-fat foods during stress: There is good evidence that these intrinsically appealing foods stimulate the brain's built-in reward system, the release of endorphins, so that you actually do feel better when you eat them. In addition, high-fat foods might be more easily eaten and digested when digestive-tract activity is suppressed by stress.

So now you know: Stress makes you eat, and when you are stressed, you prefer calorie-dense, sweet foods. I suspect that this is not a big surprise to many of you. It's not much of a surprise to most of my patients. Still, it's nice to know that it's not just you or your lack of willpower. It's a natural response to the world we live in.

On the other hand, I'm certainly not advising you to just accept that and live with it. If stress is making you eat, you have to figure out a way to reduce your stress where possible and give yourself a replacement stress-reducer for unavoidable pressure.

What can you do to reduce stress? First of all, I tell my patients that they have to learn how to say no. The only way to reduce your stress is to make more room for yourself in your life. Your needs—physical and mental—have to be put higher on your priority list. This means that other people will not always think you are perfect. Trying to be perfect for others is one of the key causes of stress in this world. You need to take care of yourself, and sometimes that means that you take care of others less.

And with the extra time you will have once you start saying no to other people's needs, you need to start doing things for yourself. They ought to be things that will help you combat the ravages of the stress you just can't avoid. Exercise has been shown to help; meditation helps; eating in a way that is good for you helps. Just about anything you can do to make your life better will help you to better deal with the stress the world forces on us.

There are stresses that can't be avoided, those that are part of your everyday life. Deadlines, for example, are common stressors; travel is another stressor that frequently gets that adrenaline and cortisol going. What can you do about these? When you know you have a stressful day or week before you, you should plan for it. Try to get your exercise in early. Take your meals with you. Try to get a good night's sleep. You need to plan for these events so that they don't take their usual toll on you and your waistline.

Bottom line: When you feel that stress-induced need to feed, go for a walk, go shopping, do something that will really make you feel good. Don't just eat, because you know in the long run it doesn't help.

## HABITUAL EATING

There are lots of reasons to eat besides being hungry or feeling upset. For example, you go out to dinner and to the movies. You buy a bag of popcorn even though you just ate. Despite the fact that you're not hungry, it tastes good and feels right. In fact, it's hard to imagine going to the movies and not eating popcorn. This is an example of eating that's triggered by something other than the experience of hunger. In this case, it is triggered by habit. You always get popcorn when you go to the movies, so even when you are not hungry, you get popcorn. If you don't, it feels odd. That's because you've made a link between these two activities, so that whenever you do the one, you want to do the other. It's one of the many ways we take in calories without even noticing.

What if you got a medium bag of popcorn with butter and a medium cola? These days that seems like a modest movie-viewing purchase. The popcorn is 500 calories (only 300 without the butter) and a 12-ounce cola is 145 calories. Without really thinking about it, you've consumed 645 calories. And you weren't even hungry!

Another common opportunity for eating without hunger is watching television. This may be the number one eating-activity pairing in the nation. It is certainly the one most solidly linked to obesity. In a recent study published in *JAMA*, researchers at Harvard followed more than 50,000 women over 6 years who were either normal weight or somewhat over the average weight. During that time, 3,800 women, just under 8 percent of them, became very overweight. When those women were compared to women who were similar in BMI, exercise level, smoking status, and diet, the primary difference between the women who gained a lot of weight and those who didn't was television. And the more television they watched, the greater their risk of getting fat.

You might think that the weight gain was just from inactivity and not specific to television, but when these researchers compared

having a sedentary job or the amount of time spent reading or playing board games, television watching created a much bigger risk for
weight gain.

Why is that? One theory is that watching television makes you
eat. Food advertising on television is ubiquitous—in a study done
more than 10 years ago, researchers noted a commercial for food
every 4 minutes. Moreover, more than 60 percent of these commercials were for high-fat, low-nutritional-value foods.

Since these women were bombarded with ads for bad foods, the
thought was that they were more likely to eat them. And, in fact, the
women in this study did report eating more calories per day with a
higher intake of high-fat, low-nutritional-value foods. There have
been studies showing similar associations between watching TV and
higher food intake in men and children, too.

Could not watching television, then, be a weight-reduction strategy? Researchers in California recently showed that by reducing the
amount of television children watched as well as the frequency of
eating in front of the television, overweight children lost weight. It
worked for them, so chances are, if you're a big-time TV watcher, it
will work for you.

Eating while watching TV might be our worst problem, but it's
not the only one. Some folks eat and read, others eat while driving.
One patient of mine has a hard time talking on the phone if she's not
nibbling on "a little something." If you eat a snack because you are
hungry, when you get to the next meal, you are less hungry, so you
eat less. But when you eat even though you aren't hungry, it doesn't
change how much you eat at your next meal. So this snack that you
are not even hungry for just adds that many more calories to what
you eat in a day, without even addressing the real issue—the real
danger in trying to lose weight—hunger.

Moreover, when you eat while you are doing something else,
you tend to eat more. This is true even if you are hungry. Reading the
paper, talking on the phone, driving—these activities distract you

from your bodies' cues that you have had enough to eat. In a series of experiments in France, researchers watched forty normal-weight women as they ate under different conditions. One meal they ate alone, with no distractions; at another meal, each ate listening to a tape of a detective story, and then, finally, they ate together in groups of four. For all the women, eating while distracted, that is, while listening to the story on tape, caused them to eat more—much more—than when they were eating alone or eating in a group.

Bottom line: Don't eat when you're not hungry—those calories taken in are the real empty ones. And when you are hungry, don't eat while you are doing something else.

# CHAPTER 14

# LIFESTYLE

## EATING OUT

If you have a score of 30 or higher in the Eating Out section, then eating away from home is likely to be a factor in your difficulty in losing weight or maintaining your weight loss.

Just 25 years ago, more than three-quarters of the food we ate was consumed at home. Now, in some age groups, almost half our food is eaten out. We are twice as likely to eat at a restaurant or fast-food joint as we used to be (from consuming around 15 percent of our calories there to just over a quarter) or from a vending machine (which has almost doubled in the same time period).

Our working life forces some of this change on us, whether we like it or not. Few of us live close enough to work to actually go home for lunch, or sometimes even for supper. And often, in this climate of pressure for higher productivity, mealtime is one of the rare occasions we have to relax and enjoy time with our colleagues and friends at work. So we can find ourselves going out to lunch virtually every day or, at the other end of the spectrum, trying to skip lunch. It seems as though our work schedules are conspiring to make us fat.

In fact, there is some evidence that they are. In a recent study from Japan, where obesity is growing almost as fast as it is here, researchers followed a large group of workers over a period of 3 years. There was a good correlation between the number of overtime hours worked and weight. The more they worked, the fatter these mostly male workers became. The researchers speculated that it was a combination of a change in eating habits (eating more meals at work rather than at home) and less time in which to exercise. The same study done here would, I suspect, reveal the same. Obviously, when eating at home, we have much more control over what we eat than we do when we eat out.

It's not just where we eat that has changed. What we eat when we do eat out has also changed dramatically—in size. When you look at the food pyramid or any of the dietary recommendations put out by nutrition agencies, amounts of food are usually described by number of servings. According to the food pyramid, we are supposed to eat 5 to 7 servings of grains, breads, or pasta per day. We're not told what that serving size should be. A serving is a serving is a serving—right? No. The FDA, the agency with the job of establishing serving sizes so that they can regulate food labels, based them on what the average serving size was when these guidelines were developed in the 1980s. What a difference a quarter of a century has made!

A recent study compared current serving sizes of commonly consumed foods that you buy when you're eating out today with those used in the food pyramid and on food labels. The difference was mind boggling. Let's just move through an ordinary day of eating out.

Say you have a bagel for breakfast. The FDA serving size is 2 ounces, but the bagel you buy at a chain bagel place like Dunkin' Donuts or Bruegger's Bagel Bakery is 4½ ounces—more than twice the bagel it used to be. If you go for a muffin, the FDA-recognized serving size is also 2 ounces. The average—this is the *average*, not the biggest—was more than three times that size, and some muffins were six times that size! That means that with one muffin, you have eaten all the grains and breads you are supposed to eat for the rest of the day! It would be okay if you knew that and adjusted for it, but who knew?

Let's move on to lunch. Say you had a hamburger; you're watching your weight, so you take a pass on the fries. The USDA figures that your burger and your bun together should be 4 ounces. Remember, though this seems small to you now, their sizes were based on the average size of the portion back in the 1980s, when the pyramid was designed. The current fast-food burger-bun combo is larger as well, at 6 ounces. And this is just the regular burger, not the Big Mac or Whopper. If you ate at a chain restaurant, like TGIF or Applebee's, that burger-bun combo is *twice* the size of the pyramid portion, at 9 ounces. That's very close to the maximum daily amount of meat recommended on the food pyramid.

Okay, how about supper? You had a burger for lunch, so you figure you'll eat light for dinner. How about some pasta? At a chain restaurant, the average serving of pasta is six times larger than the FDA allowance for a serving of pasta.

It's no wonder that our average calorie intake has increased by 600 calories a day in the past 30 years—600 calories a day! You do the math: There are 3,500 calories in a pound of fat. Increasing your calorie count by 600 calories per day means that you put on an average of a pound every 6 days! No wonder that over the past 20 years the percentage of Americans who are overweight has doubled.

Americans have recognized this change in portion size and welcomed it, although I suspect they didn't really understand what it meant to the real bottom line, the waistline. You can't accuse American business of not responding to consumer demand. They heard, and they were more than happy to oblige with huge servings of bad food.

The same supersizing trend has moved into our vending machines, too. Look at a regular chocolate candy bar. While there are big ones, the small ones look about the same to me. That's because I have a crummy memory. A Hershey bar, when it came out, had 0.6 ounce of chocolate. The small Hershey bar sold today is almost three times that size, at 1.6 ounces.

Let me remind you: Portion size is learned. How do we know this? The first evidence came from experiments on rats. In laboratories rats were given as much rat chow as they wanted. Once this portion size was determined, the rats were fed that amount daily. After a week or so of this, the portion size was increased. At first, the rats continued to eat the same amount of food, leaving the excess untouched. But after several days, the rats started eating the excess. When allowed to eat freely in an unrestricted fashion, as they had been originally, they ate this bigger portion but no more. They had learned a new portion size, which they then expected to eat at each meal.

We behave the same way as lab rats. Barbara Rolls, Ph.D., a researcher at Pennsylvania State University, decided to check this portion theory out. She recruited a group of adults and had them eat several meals. Before each meal, each person was asked to rate his hunger. Then they were served a meal. What the participants didn't know was that with each meal they were being served larger and larger portions. Despite having the same amount of hunger, these volunteers ate the larger portions. They learned a new portion size.

This is not just a laboratory phenomenon either. The same thing has happened here in the real world as well. Greg Critser, in his book *Fat Land*, suggests we've been inside a giant portion laboratory since fast-food franchises started selling more (food) for less (money) 15 years ago. It all started with Taco Bell. Some of their market research suggested that the reason people came back to their restaurants over and over and over again was not because of taste or quality but because of value and savings. So, the Taco Bell head honcho took a risk: What if he made the food an even bigger bargain? Would customers come back even more frequently?

They cut their prices and held their collective breath. The word went out and . . . business boomed. But what was really amazing— even to the executive at Taco Bell—the people who came didn't end up spending less money. Instead, they bought more food. Like the rats, when presented with more food (for the same amount of money), we might have balked initially, but in no time we ate it, enjoyed it, and finally insisted on it.

In the few short years since Taco Bell made this remarkable discovery, everybody's gotten in on the act. Value meals—under one name or the other—are ubiquitous. And it's not just in fast-food joints either. Everywhere you go, food has been supersized. Even the finest restaurants now heap food onto our plates. Name a food and the chances are that over the past decade the serving size has grown. Soft drinks are bigger; donuts are bigger; brownies are bigger; a slice of pizza is bigger; even salads are bigger.

No matter what type of diet you end up on, managing your weight requires that you scale down your portion sizes. If big portions can be learned, so can small portions. The problem is that you will be doing this on your own. Don't expect restaurants and vending machines to reduce the size of their portions. It's been way too profitable for them to reverse the trend.

Larger portion sizes in foods we eat away from home have undoubtedly contributed to the expanding American waistline, but the world we live in often makes it difficult not to eat out. What's a working stiff to do?

There are some tricks to eating out that may make it easier for you. There's no magic here, just common sense.

1. Take your lunch and snacks to work with you. When you are trying to lose weight, it's easier to control both what you eat and how much of it you eat when you make it yourself.

2. If you eat your lunch at your desk, use the extra time that you would have spent had you gone out to lunch by taking a brisk walk or exercising with your friends.

3. If you have to eat a meal out, take snacks to work so that when you do go out for lunch or supper, you're not so hungry that you inhale the bread as soon as you sit down.

4. Order one or two appetizers rather than an entrée. Often the appetizers come more quickly, so you don't have to wait as long to eat. You'll be surprised at how much they fill you up. Appetizers have also grown, and often, what is now considered an appetizer size used to be a whole serving.

5. Order a half size or appetizer size of a pasta or other entrée. If the restaurant doesn't do that, ask the server to bring you only half and pack the rest up for you to take home, or split the dish with a friend.

6. Send away the bread before it even lands on the table.

7. Don't hesitate to tell the server how you would like your food prepared. If you want it broiled rather than fried or with the sauce on the side, ask for it that way. A restaurant would rather let you "have it your way" and come back again than not.

8. Find the restaurants in your area that serve foods that you can eat on your diet. A fat-counting diet is the hardest to pursue when eating out, because restaurants add fats to just about everything to improve flavor and appearance.

9. Get all sauces served on the side.

10. Eat the foods that you'll feel good about eating first. Save the higher-calorie foods for last. When you get a steak and salad, eat the salad first.

11. Avoid drinking an alcoholic beverage before your meal, and limit your alcohol consumption during a meal.

12. When you know you are going to be dining out, allow for the extra calories you will undoubtedly consume by being selective in what you eat before and after your restaurant meal.

13. When you overeat, forgive yourself and get back on the diet—before you add insult to injury by eating dessert, too.

One last point: Many of my patients have told me that when they go out to eat with their friends and order just an appetizer or a salad, they worry that their friends perceive this as an assault on their eating habits, since they are ordering the usual big lunch. I suspect that this is true some of the time. But the world we live in is pushing us down the path to obesity. If you want to get off that path, it's going to make you different. Here's your choice: You can continue with them on their path and end up with the same weight problems as your friends, or you can find your own way to the weight you want.

Sometimes others may feel that the choices you make for yourself imply a criticism about them. It's not that. You know that as well as I do. Their feelings are a projection of their own concerns about their weight. They have to make their own choices. You must be free to make yours.

## DAILY ACTIVITY

A score of 60 or less in the Daily Activity part of the questionnaire indicates that your activity level is contributing to your difficulty in maintaining the weight you want. In many polls, 60 percent of Americans have acknowledged that they are mostly sedentary. That's what they admit to. Here's what we know about physical activity: It makes you feel better and live longer, it helps you lose weight and maintain weight loss once you've achieved your ideal weight, and you don't have to exercise to get the benefits that physical activity has to offer. If physical activity isn't exercise, what is it? Basically, it's anything you do that requires you to move. Many of us live our lives in an environment that only asks us to walk from the house to the car, then a few steps from the car to the office, and spend the rest of the day sitting, except for a few steps to the bathroom and lunch room and then back to the car.

Physical activity is anything we do that is more than that. Walking down the hall to communicate with a colleague rather than just sending a quick e-mail. Parking in the far lot to add a brisk walk to each end of your day. Walking the kids to school rather than driving. A recent study showed that folks who live in an urban setting tend to be thinner than those who live in the suburbs. Why is that? Because urbanites have to walk more than their suburban counterparts.

Researchers in the 1990s looked at physical activity and saw that much of the cardiovascular benefit accrued even when the activity was not vigorous and didn't last half an hour. And, of course, any activity will burn calories.

A study done a few years ago compared the weight-loss benefit of increasing daily activity versus adding an exercise regimen in response to the traditional recommendation to exercise more. Several thousand sedentary, overweight adults were divided into two groups. Both groups were instructed to follow a weight-reduction diet, and one group was instructed to exercise for 30 minutes per day. The other was counseled to increase their everyday activity by walking up stairs, parking a couple of blocks from work, and standing rather than sitting.

Initially, the group instructed to exercise lost more weight, but after two years the two groups had evened out. In fact, more folks in the activity group were getting 30 minutes of exercise at least three times per week than in the exercise group. Moreover, in both groups, the individuals who were more active reported more weight loss and feeling better overall.

So even if you hate the gym, can't stand sweating, wouldn't work out if your life depended on it, you can increase the amount of activity in your life and reap many of the benefits of exercising without actually having to do it.

## WHAT CAN YOU DO?

1. Take the stairs rather than the elevator. One flight of stairs can burn off 10 calories. You might think that's not much, but if you did a couple of flights every day, it adds up.

2. Don't drive all the way to work. Park a couple of blocks away and walk the difference. If you walk one-fifth of a mile, about four blocks, you burn off 20 to 25 calories. Do it both ways, and you're making a difference.

3. Try standing while you watch television. Standing for an hour burns 10 to 20 calories. Pacing can also help. You burn off a calorie with each 15 steps taken.

4. If you have a sit-down job, think up reasons to get up and walk. Rather than e-mail a colleague, walk over to his office and see him. Rather than send something by interoffice mail, take it yourself.

5. Take a short walk every day before lunch. It will make your lunch taste better, and a brisk 15- to 20-minute walk can burn off 100 calories.

6. Find businesses close to your home or office, and walk there when you do errands instead of driving there.

7. Keep track of your activity. Anything you do that has you moving can be counted as activity. On the opposite page is a list of activities and the calories you burn doing them for just 10 minutes. See if you can increase the calories you burn by just a few calories per day.

## EXERCISE

If you have a score of 2 or less in the Exercise section of the questionnaire, then you probably are having some difficulty getting yourself to work out. Here's the problem with that: Without exercise, you dramatically reduce the likelihood that you will be able to maintain your weight loss. It's as simple as that. Let me remind you of the good that exercise provides.

# CALORIES BURNED IN EVERYDAY ACTIVITIES

| Activity | Calories Burned in 10 Minutes Body weight: 125 | Calories Burned in 10 Minutes Body weight: 175 |
|---|---|---|
| Bicycling (5.5 mph) | 42 | 58 |
| Carpentry | 32 | 44 |
| Chopping wood | 60 | 84 |
| Dancing (moderate) | 35 | 48 |
| Dressing or washing | 26 | 37 |
| House painting | 29 | 40 |
| Light gardening | 30 | 42 |
| Light office work | 25 | 34 |
| Making beds | 32 | 46 |
| Mowing the grass (using power mower) | 34 | 47 |
| Ping-pong | 32 | 45 |
| Preparing food | 32 | 46 |
| Shoveling snow | 65 | 90 |
| Sitting (watching TV) | 10 | 14 |
| Sitting and talking | 15 | 21 |
| Sleeping | 10 | 14 |
| Standing | 12 | 15 |
| Standing (light activity) | 20 | 28 |
| Walking (2 mph) | 29 | 40 |
| Walking (4 mph) | 52 | 72 |
| Walking downstairs | 56 | 78 |
| Walking upstairs | 146 | 202 |
| Washing floors | 35 | 48 |
| Weeding | 49 | 68 |

1. It burns off calories, which allows you to eat a few more goodies than you would be able to without exercise.

2. It reduces stress and improves symptoms of anxiety and depression.

3. It decreases mortality.

4. It makes your body feel better.

5. It makes your body look better.

6. It reduces your appetite (in the long run).

7. It makes you think more clearly.

8. Exercise is absolutely the only thing you can do that will really increase your metabolism and allow you to burn off more calories even when you sleep.

So what are the barriers to exercise? They are as many and diverse as we are. While how much we eat has increased, the amount of activity in our lives has decreased. Although the vast majority of Americans describe themselves as sedentary, I would argue that we are not sedentary because we are lazy. We were not built to be sedentary, but the way our world is structured right now makes it hard not to be. You have to work—sometimes very hard—in order to restore a natural level of activity to life.

In most places in this country, you could take a walk, but where would you go? You usually can't just walk to the store: It's miles away. And frequently, there are no sidewalks to give us a place to walk, no crosswalks to get us across the streets safely. Where we live and work has been designed to accommodate cars. And there is good in that: We don't have to walk to the store to get milk in the pouring rain or snow, but it has also made the normal activity level necessary to get through the day remarkably small. A woman now spends 400 calories less in a single day's activity than a woman at the start of the twentieth century. We are not hauling water or scrubbing floors on our knees or bringing in wood to keep the home fires burning. And thank God. Believe me, I am not advocating a return to earlier times. But what this means is that activity, the natural exercise we are all designed for, has been taken out of the realm of everyday life and now has to be put back intentionally.

That can feel fake and somewhat silly. When you are busy, it can seem dopey to walk to the store or to cycle to work, when it's just faster and more efficient to drive. And taking the stairs rather than the elevator can often appear an odd choice, especially since the stairs are frequently dark and dirty and hard to find. Then, after working a full day and taking care of everyone at home, we are expected to choose to spend our rare free time exercising? It seems an unreasonable choice to many, and so we live in a country where most people are sedentary.

And yet, the physical, mental, and psychological benefits of exercise are undeniable. The first reason I get from my patients as to why they are not exercising is that they don't have time. And many of my patients have families, which means that they work a job and then come home and work that second unpaid job. There is no doubt that these people are very busy.

The second reason offered by most of my patients is that they don't like to exercise. I suspect that is really the reason that most of us don't exercise. We just haven't found a way to do it that feels good and is enjoyable.

But we must.

I can't promise you that you will achieve your ideal weight. I can't promise you that you will have the body you so long for. But here is a promise I feel 100 percent comfortable making: If you exercise, you will feel better. Period.

Our bodies are designed to move, even when they are out of shape and overweight. If you move, your body will feel better and so will the rest of you. The trick, I think, is to find some way to move that suits you that you can incorporate into your everyday life.

First, let's think about what you don't like about exercise. Well, there's the whole time thing: It's just one more thing that you have to incorporate into an already busy life. That's true. We all live very busy, stressful lives, and it's hard to imagine shoving one more thing into them. But who takes care of the caretaker? If you spend your days taking care of others, as so many of us do, you need to make time and space for yourself in order to keep up that caretaking.

Lily Tomlin said something really wise in one of her monologues: "For fast-acting relief, try slowing down." Slow down; take some time for yourself, even if it means doing less for others. One of the reasons my patients don't do this is because they want others to think that they are perfect: perfectly competent and capable; perfectly able to take care of everything. The only one they can stint on, if that is their goal, is themselves. And they do it. Frequently.

So, make time for yourself. You make time for others. Are you a morning person? Get up half an hour earlier and use that time to exercise. Are you a night owl? Stay up a little later and use the extra time to exercise.

Another barrier to exercise is lack of experience. Many Americans have never exercised, or at least not in a long, long time. Because it's been so long, they don't remember the good feeling they got after exercising. Trust me—it's there.

The fear of not being good at something is another hurdle. We're out of the habit of learning new things, many of us. We're uneasy at the prospect of looking like a beginner. So, why not start by doing something you already know how to do? The most popular exercise is walking, and that's a perfect place to start.

Some people don't want to be seen exercising. They are embarrassed about their bodies or their physical skills. Do something you can do at home. Get an exercise video and work out along with that. Get a treadmill. Get an exercise bike. Secondhand, barely used exercise machines are a dime a dozen. And if you decide to exercise at home, go out of your way to make it a pleasant experience. No one will use a stationary bike in the basement. Do your exercises in a pleasant environment, and make an effort to maximize the pleasure you get from them. Do you think walking on a treadmill is dull? Then do it in front of the TV set. Or listen to books on tape or to music. Try to make it fun. Starting to exercise takes a certain amount of what chemistry calls "activation energy." It takes more energy to get started, but once you do, it's not nearly as hard to continue. Remember that when you are lying in bed, trying to think of good reasons not to get up and out.

Finally, I think many of my patients have very little experience with the huge variety available in exercise. They have tried running or walking or cycling and didn't like it, so their conclusion is that they don't like exercise. Keep trying. Find the exercise you enjoy and then stick to it. It will pay off. Don't be afraid to try different exercises. How about yoga? Or tai chi? Pilates? Dance workouts? Be creative. Find something you like and stick with it.

When you start off, start slow and low. If you haven't really exercised in quite a long time, you can start by doing just 10 minutes. After a few weeks, add another 10 minutes. It doesn't have to be 20 minutes at a stretch; 10 and 10 work just as well.

And you don't have to exercise until you "feel the burn," as Jane Fonda used to say. The way you gauge the effort you are expending is to measure your pulse. The faster your heart is beating, the harder you are working. But the best way to burn fat is not by working the hardest—the hardest work is good for your heart. But the best speed to burn off fat is much lower, and that's good news to many of us.

Here's how to determine your target heart rate. For starters, get a calculator; you'll need it.

To calculate the rate for burning fat, subtract your age from 220:

220 − _____ = _____

Multiply that by 0.65:

_____ × 0.65 = _____ beats per minute

That number is your target heart rate when you want to burn fat.

For a cardiovascular workout, again subtract your age from 220:

$$220 - \underline{\hspace{2cm}} = \underline{\hspace{2cm}}$$

This time multiply that number by 0.85:

$$\underline{\hspace{2cm}} \times 0.85 = \underline{\hspace{2cm}} \text{ beats per minute}$$

I usually check my pulse at my carotid artery. It is located just under the angle of your jaw on your neck. It's not easy to miss. I count for 10 seconds and then multiply that number by 6 to get the beats per minute.

Many of my patients who finally fell in love with exercise started by exercising with a friend. It tends to keep you honest and motivated. You and your buddy can take turns being the lazy one and the energetic one. And it's a great way to make exercise a little more fun, and that's particularly important at the beginning. After you have started walking, cycling, swimming, or whatever you decide works for you, you need to consider adding weight lifting, or resistance training, to the program. Weight lifting builds muscle better than any other activity. The more muscle you have, the higher your metabolism. The higher your metabolism, the more calories you burn in your sleep.

In weight or resistance training, how you do it—form—is the most important thing. So, consider getting a few lessons from a weight trainer in your area. You don't have to join a gym; you can do this stuff at home, but you need to do it correctly.

How much exercise do you need? Less than you might think. The official recommendation is 30 minutes a day for most days of the week. If you aim for 150 minutes per week, I think you'll find that's a good starting point. Recent research shows that with exercise more is just more. People who have lost weight and kept it off exercise for an average of 210 minutes per week. That is 30 minutes, 7 days a week. That should be your goal.

Pay attention to your body and try to have fun. Here's my promise again. If you exercise, you *will* feel better.

# AFTERWORD

*"To eat is a necessity, but to eat intelligently is an art."*
—François La Rochefoucauld, Maxims 1665

The goal of this book has been to teach you the art of eating intelligently. Only by eating wisely will we be able to manage our weight in a world that eagerly and aggressively seeks to fatten us up. To achieve this wisdom, we need to combine what science has to teach us about eating and exercise with what we know about ourselves. Of these two, I would say that self-knowledge is the most important. Nevertheless, in this book I have aspired to provide you with the tools to acquire both.

The questionnaire will help you understand the hows and whys of the ways you eat. This knowledge will help you to identify the characteristics of your diet—the one you developed over your life-time of eating—and with that knowledge you can begin to under-stand what can be changed and what cannot. The information about the nutrition and physiology of eating will guide you to making choices about the diet and lifestyle you need to stay healthy and fit for the rest of your life.

Of course, the questionnaire and the research on nutrition and diet provide a snapshot of two very dynamic processes. Inevitably both will change over time. It's easiest to see in the context of your own life: You get a new job, and—boom—you're spending lots more time at work. It's suddenly hard to find time to exercise (again). Your diet seems to spin out of control (again) as you eat your way through lunch after lunch with new colleagues and contacts. Or maybe you have a baby, and not only do you have to lose weight (again), your life is suddenly a lot more complicated.

Nor does it take life-altering events like these to change the choices you've made about diet and exercise. What happens if you get injured while running? What happens if your treadmill breaks or your gym goes out of business? All of these events will require you to go back and revisit some of the same issues you're dealing with now. Your diet and lifestyle are constantly changing. You need to take charge of those changes and make sure they work for you and your goals. My aim has been to help you recognize patterns in how you eat and live so you can use that understanding to manage your weight. Knowing not only what you eat and do but *why* you do them will help you make choices you can live with.

The science of diet will change, too, no doubt. We are at the threshold of a very exciting time in this field. Research scientists and physicians are flocking to this growing area of inquiry. The future will bring new discoveries about how the foods and drugs we put into our bodies work in combination with the genes passed on to us by our parents, in the world we have to live in. These discoveries should make it easier for us to understand how our choices affect us, now and in the future.

In the meantime, however, I have tried to give you enough information so that when your life changes, you'll understand how you can adapt to those changes. This book, I hope, will be your toolbox when life changes necessitate lifestyle change.

Finally, you may be wondering, why is all this necessary? Until very recently we didn't need books telling us how to eat and live in order to be healthy. Why now? We are facing a world that has changed in a very fundamental way. Never before has a single population had access to so much food in so much variety and at such a small cost. And never before has the livin' been quite so easy for so many of us.

Too much of our available abundance consists of high-calorie foods that make us fat without necessarily making us full. Agribusiness has been extremely successful: We grow a quantity and variety of foods that would have been unimaginable even 50 years ago.

Because of that incredible success, the overfeeding of America may well have been unavoidable, at least from a business point of view. Companies that make and sell food, like companies that make and sell just about anything—computers, DVD players, sneakers— prosper by selling us more. The problem is that their market, the food buyers of America, is not growing, at least not fast enough. Innovations in agribusiness have allowed food producers to make available to us 3,800 calories per day, 700 more than were produced just 30 years ago. In order to maintain profits and continued growth, food companies set out to do what any business would do: Persuade each of us to buy—and eat—more, a lot more. And we have.

In supermarkets, on the road, on television, the message is clear and practically continuous: Eat! Eat! Eat! Our bodies were built to withstand the stresses of starvation. In confronting this new stress, the stress of overabundance, we are naked and virtually defenseless, evolutionarily speaking. When the invitation to eat and eat and eat is extended, genetically we are programmed to say yes, yes, yes. But in this environment of plenty, that answer has made us what we are today: one of the fattest nations in the world.

We need to develop strategies to navigate through this new and very different threat. In the distant past, this was the job of genes.

More recently, culture has helped us choose the foods that made us survive. But those defenses have been outpaced by the rapid changes that mark this time in our history. They may catch up, but genes exert their influence over millennia, and culture over centuries. So we have to figure out our own strategy right now if we want to retain control over our health and well-being. And the only tool we have is education and a willingness to take charge of the way we live and eat.

We are not helpless creatures facing a dangerous world over which we have no control. The choices we make in the marketplace will be heard and felt. City hall and industry can respond to the demands of their constituents and customers. There is a growing movement in this country to change the toxic environment that has pushed us to become one of the fattest nations in the world. But that kind of change takes time, too, and many of us just can't wait.

The world we live in makes eating intelligently a necessity as well as an art. Making the choices that are right for each of us is our best hope of shaping the lives and bodies we want. This book, I hope, will make that difficult goal just a little easier.

# BIBLIOGRAPHY

## BOOKS

I reviewed hundreds of articles and books in the writing of this book. I have listed the most important references and those that will be most easily found and understood by my readers. These are books and resources that I depended on throughout the writing of this book. These contain information and ideas that so informed the fundamentals of this book that ideas and information from or derived from them appear on practically every page. These I have listed separately. Specific references are listed afterward by chapter.

## Selected Bibliography

Berne, R.M., and M.N. Levy. *The Principles of Physiology.* St. Louis: The CV Mosby Company, 1990.

Brownell, Kelly D. *The LEARN Program for Weight Management 2000.* Dallas, TX: American Health Publishing Company, 2000.

Clinical guidelines on the identification, evaluation, and treatment of overweight and obesity in adults: The evidence report/National Heart, Lung, and Blood Institute in cooperation with the National Institute of Diabetes and Digestive and Kidney Disease. Bethesda, Maryland: National Institutes of Health, National Heart, Lung, and Blood Institute, 1998.

*Clinical Obesity*, edited by Peter G. Kopelman and Michael J. Stock. Oxford; Malden, Massachusetts: Blackwell Sciences, 1998.

Crister, Greg. *Fat Land: How Americans became the fattest people in the world.* Boston: Houghton Mifflin, 2003.

Katz, David. *Nutrition in Clinical Practice.* Philadelphia: Lippincott, Williams and Wilkins, 2001.

Mann, Jim, and Stewart Truswell. *Essentials of Human Nutrition.* New York: Oxford University Press, 1998.

Nestle, Marion. *Food Politics: How the food industry influences nutrition and health.* Berkeley, California: University of California Press, 2002.

Peake, P. *Fight Fat After 40.* New York: Penguin, 2001.

Willett, Walter C. *Eat Drink and Be Healthy.* New York: Simon & Schuster, 2001.

All nutritional values for foods were taken from *The Nutribase Nutrition Facts Desk Reference*. Avery, New York, 2001.

## 1: There Is a Prefect Diet for Everyone

Bravata, D.M., L. Sanders, J. Huang, H.M. Krumholz, I. Olkin, and C.D. Gardner. "Efficacy and safety of low-carbohydrate diets: A systematic review." *Journal of the American Medical Association,* 289 (2003): 1837–50.

Bartoshuk, L.M., V.B. Duffy, L.A. Lucchina, J. Prutkin, and K. Fast. "Supertasters and the saltiness of salt," *Annals of the New York Academy of Sciences,* 855 (1998): 793–96.

Kim, U., E. Jorgenson, H. Coon, M. Leppert, N. Risch, and D. Drayna. "Positional cloning of the human quantitative trait locus underlying taste sensitivity to phenylthiocarbamide." *Science,* 299 (2003): 1221–25.


## 2: Why One Size Doesn't Fit All

Evans, W.E., and H.L. McLeod. "Drug therapy: Pharmacogenomics—Drug disposition, drug targets, and side effects." *New England Journal of Medicine,* 348, 6 (2003): 538–49.

Weinshilboum, R. "Genomic medicine: Inheritance and drug response." *New England Journal of Medicine,* 348, 6 (2003): 529–37.

Materson, B.J., D.J. Reda, W.C. Cushman, et al. "Single-drug therapy for hypertension in men—A comparison of six antihypertensive agents with placebo." *New England Journal of Medicine,* 328 (1999): 914–21.

Bouchard, C., Tremblay, A., Despres, J.P., et al. "The response to long-term overfeeding in identical twins." *New England Journal of Medicine,* 322 (1990): 1477–82.

Hainer, V., A.J. Stunkard, M. Kunesova, J. Parizkova, V. Stich, and D.B. Allison. "Intrapair resemblance in very low calorie diet-induced weight loss in female obese identical twins." *International Journal of Obesity & Related Metabolic Disorders,* 24, 8 (2000): 1051–57.

Kopp W. "High-insulinogenic nutrition—anetiologic factor for obesity and the metabolic syndrome?" *Metabolism*, 52, 7 (2003): 840–44.

Parks, E.J., and M.K. Hellerstein. "Carbohydrate-induced hypertriglyceridemia: Historical perspective and biological mechanisms." *American Journal of Clinical Nutrition*, 71 (2000): 412–33.

Yancy, William S. Jr., M.D., Eric C. Westman, M.D., Patricia A. French, BS, and Robert M. Califf, M.D. "Diets and clinical coronary events: The truth is out there." *Circulation*, 107, 1 (2003): 10–16.

Rolls, B.J. "Sensory-Specific Satiety." *Nutritional Reviews*, 44 (1966): 93–101.

Snoek, H.M., L. Huntjens, L.J. van Gemert, C. de Graaf, and H. Weener. "Sensory-specific satiety in obese and normal-weight women." *American Journal of Clinical Nutrition*, 80, 4 (2004): 823–31.

Rolls, B.J., E.A. Bell, and B.A. Waugh. "Increasing the volume of a food by incorporating air affects satiety in men." *American Journal of Clinical Nutrition*, 72 (2000): 361–68.

Burton-Freeman, B., P.A. Davis, and B.O. Schneeman. "Plasma cholecystokinin is associated with subjective measures of satiety in women." *American Journal of Clinical Nutrition*, 76, 3 (2002): 659–67.

Aksyonov, Vassily. *In Search of Melancholy Baby.* New York: Random House, 1987.

## 3: How the Perfect Fit Diet Works

Haines, P.S., M.Y. Hama, D.K. Guilkey, and B.M. Popkin. "Weekend eating in the United States is linked with greater energy, fat, and alcohol intake." *Obesity Research*, 11 (2003): 945–49.

Schoeller, D.A. "How accurate is self-reported dietary energy intake?" *Nutritional Review*, 48 (1990): 373–79.

Lichtman, S.W., et al. "Discrepancy between self-reported and actual caloric intake and exercise in obese subjects." *New England Journal of Medicine,* 327 (1992): 1893–98.

Marmonier, C., D. Chapelot, and J. Louis-Sylvestre. "Metabolic and behavioral consequences of a snack consumed in a satiety state." *American Journal of Clinical Nutrition,* 70, 5 (1999): 854–66.

Marmonier C., D. Chapelot, M. Fantino, and J. Louis-Sylvestre. "Snacks consumed in a nonhungry state have poor satiating efficiency: Influence of snack composition on substrate utilization and hunger." *American Journal of Clinical Nutrition,* 76, 3 (2002): 518–28.

Sanders, L., D. Bravata, K. Page, and M. Brainerd. "Diets and exercise programs for weight loss." *Nutritional Health,* Totowa, New Jersey: Humana Press, 2005.

Story, M., and P. Faulkner. "The prime time diet: A content analysis of eating behavior and food messages in television program content and commercials." *American Journal of Public Health,* 80, 6 (1990): 738–40.

## 4: Getting Started

Lichtman, S.W., et al. "Discrepancy between self-reported and actual caloric intake and exercise in obese subjects." *New England Journal of Medicine,* 327 (1992): 1893–98.

Day, N.E., McKeown, M.Y. Wong, A. Welch, and S. Bingham. "Epidemiological assesment of diet: A comparison of a 7 day diary with a food frequency questionnaire using urinary markers of nitrogen, potassium and sodium." *International Journal of Epidemiology,* 80 (2001): 309–17.

Goris, A.H.C., M.S. Westerterp-Plantegna, and K.R. Westerterp. "Undereating and underrecording of habitual food intake in obese men: Selective underreporting of fat intake." *American Journal of Clinical Nutrition,* 71 (2000): 130–34.

## 6: The Counting Carbohydrates Diet

Ludwig, D.S. "The glycemic index: Physiological mechanisms relating to obesity, diabetes, and cardiovascular disease." *Journal of the American Medical Association*, 287 (2002): 2414–23.

Ebbeling, C.B., M.M. Leidig, K.B. Sinclair, J.P. Hangen, and D.S. Ludwig. "A reduced-glycemic load diet in the treatment of adolescent obesity." *Archaeological Pediatrician Adolescent Medicine*, 157 (August 2003): 773–79.

Brehm, B.J., R.J. Seeley, S.R. Daniels, and D.A. D'Alessio. "A randomized trial comparing a very low carbohydrate diet and a calorie-restricted low fat diet on body weight and cardiovascular risk factors in healthy women." *Journal of Clinical Endocrine Metabolism*, 88 (2003): 1617–23.

Yancy, W.S., M.K. Olsen, J.R. Guyton, R.P. Bakst, and E.C. Westman. "A low-carbohydrate, ketogenic diet versus a low-fat diet to treat obesity and hyperlipidemia." *Annual International Medicine* 140 (2004): 769–77.

Samaha, F.F., N.P. Iqbal, P. Seshadri, et al. "A low-carbohydrate as compared with a low-fat diet in severe obesity." *New England Journal of Medicine*, 348 (2003): 2074–81.

Stern, L., N. Iqbal, P. Seshadri, et al. "The effects of low-carbohydrate versus conventional weight loss diets in severely obese adults: One-year follow-up of a randomized trial." *Annual International Medicine*, 140 (2004): 778–85.

## 7: The Counting Calories Diet

Gutzwiller, J.P., J. Drewe, S. Ketterer, P. Hildebrand, A. Krautheim, and C. Beglinger. "Interaction between CCK and a preload on reduction of food intake is mediated by CCK-A receptors in humans." *American Journal of Physiology: Regulatory, Integrative, and Comparative Physiology*, 279 (2000): R189–95.

Stacher, G. "Satiety effects of cholecystokinin and ceruletide in lean and obese men." *Annals of the New York Academy of Sciences*, 448, 1 (1985): 431–36.

Knight, E.L., et al. "The impact of protein intake on renal function decline in women with normal renal function or mild renal insufficiency." *Annals of Internal Medicine*, 138 (2003): 460–67.

Skov, A.R., S. Toubro, J. Bulow, K. Krabbe, H.H. Parving, and A. Astrup. "Changes in renal function during weight loss induced by high vs low-protein low-fat diets in overweight subjects." *International Journal of Obesity*, 23, 11 (1999): 1170–77.

## 8: The Counting Fats Diet

Taubes, Gary. "What if it has all been a big fat lie." *The New York Times Magazine*, July 7, 2002.

Wyatt, H.R., G.K. Grunwald, C.L. Mosca, et al. "Long-term weight loss and breakfast in subjects in the National Weight Control Registry." *Obesity Research*, 10 (2002): 78–82.

Wing, R.R., and J.O. Hill. "Successful weight loss maintenance." *Annual Review of Nutrition*, 21 (2001): 323–41.

Pirozzo, S., C. Summerbell, C. Cameron, and P. Glasziou. "Advice on low-fat diets for obesity." *The Cochrane Library*, 3 (2005).

Bray, G.A., and B. Popkin. "Dietary fat intake does affect obesity." *American Journal of Clinical Nutrition*, 68 (1998): 1157–73.

Layman, D.K., R.A. Boileau, D.J. Erickson, J.E. Painter, et al. "A reduced ratio of dietary carbohydrate to protein improves body composition and blood lipid profiles during weight loss in adult women." *Journal of Nutrition*, 133 (2003): 411–17.

Rolls, B.J., V.H. Castellanos, J.C. Halford, et al. "Volume of food consumed affects satiety in men." *American Journal of Clinical Nutrition*, 67 (1998): 1170–77.

## 9: Food Preferences

### Carnimore

Skov, Annebeth R., Nikolaj Haulrik, et al. "Effect of protein intake on bone mineralization during weight loss: A 6-month trial." *Obesity Research,* 10 (2002): 432–38.

Willett, W. *Eat, Drink and Be Healthy: The Harvard Medical School Guide to Healthy Eating.* New York: Free Press, 2002

### Milk Mavin

The Honolulu Heart Program. Abbott, Robert D., Ph.D., J. David Curb, M.D., et al. "Effect of dietary calcium and milk consumption on risk of thromboembolic stroke in older middle-aged men." *Stroke,* 27 (1996): 813–18.

Skov, Annebeth R., Nikolaj Haulrik, et al. "Effect of protein intake on bone mineralization during weight loss: A 6-month trial." *Obesity Research,* 10 (2002): 432–38.

Murphy, S., K.T. Khaw, H. May, and J. E. Compston. "Milk consumption and bone mineral density in middle aged and elderly women." *British Medical Journal,* 308 (April 9, 1994): 939–41.

Davies, K. M., R. P. Heaney, R. R. Recker, J. M. Lappe, M. J. Barger-Lux, K. Rafferty, and S. Hinders. "Calcium intake and body weight." *Journal of Clinical Endocrine Metabolism,* 85 (2000): 4635–38.

Fisher, Jennifer Orlet, D. C. Mitchell, et al. "Maternal milk consumption predicts the tradeoff between milk and soft drinks in young girls' diets." *Journal of Nutrition,* 131 (2001): 246–50.

### VegeCarian

Schatzkin, Arthur, Elaine Lanza, et al. "Lack of effect of a low-fat, high-fiber diet on the recurrence of colorectal adenomas."

*New England Journal of Medicine,* 342, 16 (April 20, 2000): 1149–55.

Ludwig, D. S. "Glycemic index: History and overview." *American Journal of Clinical Nutrition* (2002): 266S–73S.

Slabber, M., et al. "Effects of a low insulin response energy restricted diet on weight loss and plasma insulin concentrations in hyperinsulinemic obese females." *American Journal Clinical of Nutrition,* 60 (1994): 48–53.

Bouche C., et al. Unpublished observation 2000, cited in J. C. Brand Miller, et al., "Glycemic index and obesity." *American Journal Clinical of Nutrition* (2002): 281S–5S.


## Sweets Eater

Levine, S., and D.T.M. Weldon, Grace, et al. "Naloxone blocks that portion of feeding driven by sweet taste in food-restricted rats." *American Journal of Physiology: Regulatory, Integrative, and Comparative Physiology,* 268, 1 (1995).

Drewnowski, A., D. D. Krahn, M. A. Demitrack, K. Nairn, and B. A. Gosnell. "Naloxone, an opiate blocker, reduces the consumption of sweet high-fat foods in obese and lean female binge eaters." *American Journal of Clinical Nutrition,* 61 (1995): 1206–12.

McCrory, M. A., et al. "Dietary variety within food groups: Association with energy intake and body fatness in men and women." *American Journal of Clinical Nutrition,* 69, 3 (1999): 440–47.

Nadeau, J., et al. "Teaching subjects with type 2 diabetes how to incorporate sugar choices into their daily meal plan promotes dietary compliance and does not deteriorate metabolic profile." *Diabetes Care,* 24, 2 (2001): 222–27.

Pelchat, M. L. "Food cravings in young and elderly adults." *Appetite,* 28, 2 (1997): 103–13.

## Waterless Wonder

Lars Breimer. Letter: "Coffee drinking was compared with tea drinking in monozygotic twins in eighteenth century." *British Medical Journal*, 312 (June 15, 1996): 1539.

Sevrens, Lyon J. "A soda a day ups the risk." *Philadelphia Daily News*, November 10, 2004.

Westerterp-Plantenga, M.S., and C.R.T. Verwegen. "The appetizing effect of an apéritif in overweight and normal-weight humans." *American Journal of Clinical Nutrition*, 69, 2 (1999): 205–12.

## PROP Taster

Atwood, Liz. "A talent for tasting: Supertasters' discriminating abilities are right on the tips of their tongues." *The Baltimore Sun*, September 29, 2004.

## 10: Dieting History

Critser, Greg. *Fat land: How Americans became the fattest people in the world*. Boston: Houghton Mifflin, 2003.

Rolls, B.J., E.L. Morris, and S.L. Roe. "Portion size of food affects energy intake in normal-weight and overweight men and women." *American Journal of Clinical Nutrition*, 76, 6 (2002): 1207–13.

Linne, Y., B. Barkeling, S. Rossner, and P. Rooth. "Vision and eating behavior." *Obesity Research*, 10, 2 (2002): 92–95.

Rolls, B.J., and E.T. Rolls, E.A. Rowe, K. Sweeney. "Sensory-specific satiety in man." *Physiology and Behavior*, 27 (1981): 137–42.

Burton-Freeman, B., P.A. Davis, and B.O. Schneeman. "Plasma cholecystokinin is associated with subjective measures of satiety in women." *American Journal of Clinical Nutrition*, 76, 3 (2002): 659–67.

Stacher, G. "Satiety effects of cholecystokinin and ceruletide in lean and obese men." *Annals of the New York Academy of Sciences*, 448, 1 (1985): 431–36.

Lieverse, R. J., J. B. Jansen, P. A. Masclee, and C. B. Lamers. "Satiety effects of a physiological dose of cholecystokinin in humans." *Gut*, 36, (1995): 176–79.

Hays, N. P., G. B. Bathalon, M. A. McCrory, et al. "Eating behavior correlates of adult weight gain and obesity in healthy women aged 55–65." *American Journal of Clinical Nutrition*, 75, 3 (2002): 476–83.

## 11: Medical History

Stefanick, M. L., Ph.D., et al. "Effects of diet and exercise in men and postmenopausal women with low levels of HDL cholesterol and high levels of LDL cholesterol." *New England Journal of Medicine*, 339, 1 (July 2, 1998): 12–20.

de Lorgeril, M., P. Salen, J.L. Martin, et al. "Mediterranean diet, traditional risk factors, and the rate of cardiovascular complications after myocardial infarction." *Circulation*, 99 (1999): 779–85.

Crapo, P. A., G. Reaven, et al. "Postprandial plasma-glucose and insulin responses to different complex carbohydrates." *Diabetes*, 26, 12 (1977): 1178–83.

McLaughlin, T., F. Abbasi, H. S. Kim, C. Lamendola, P. Schaaf, and G. Reaven. "Relationship between insulin resistance, weight loss, and coronary heart disease risk in healthy, obese women." *Metabolism*, 50, 7 (2001): 795–800.

Banz, W. J., M. A. Maher, W. G. Thompson, et al. "Effects of resistance versus aerobic training on coronary artery disease risk factors." *Experimental Biology & Medicine*, 228, 4 (2003): 434–40.

Diabetes Prevention Program Research Group "Reduction in the incidence of type 2 diabetes with lifestyle intervention or Metformin." *New England Journal of Medicine*, 346 (2002): 393–403.

Whelton, P.K., et al. "Primary prevention of hypertension: Clinical and public health advisory from the national high blood pressure education program." *Journal of the American Medical Association*, 288, 15 (2002): 1882–88.

## 12: Family Heritage

Stunkard, A.J. "An adoption study of human obesity." *New England Journal of Medicine*, 314 (1986): 193–98.

Stunkard, A.J., et al. "The body mass index of twins who have been reared apart." *New England Journal of Medicine*, 322, 21 (1990): 1483–87.

van den Bree, M.B.M., et al. "Genetic and environmental influences on eating patterns of twins aged 50 years." *American Journal of Clinical Nutrition*, 70, 4 (1999): 456–65.

Steinle, N.I., W. Hsueh, S. Snitker, et al. "Eating behavior in the Old Order Amish: Heritability analysis and a genome-wide linkage analysis." *American Journal of Clinical Nutrition*, 75 (2002): 1098–1106.

## 13: Eating Habits

Ortega, R.M., et al. "Associations between obesity, breakfast-time food habits and intake of energy and nutrients in a group of elderly Madrid residents." *Journal of the American College of Nutrition*, 15 (1996): 65–72.

Levine, A.S., et al. "Effect of breakfast cereals on short-term food intake." *American Journal of Clinical Nutrition*, 50 (1989): 1303–07.

Schlundt, D.G., et al. "The role of breakfast in the treatment of obesity: a randomized clinical trial." *American Journal of Clinical Nutrition*, 55 (1992): 645–51.

Wyatt, H.R., G.K. Grunwald, C.L. Mosca, et al. "Long-term weight loss and breakfast in subjects in the National Weight Control Registry." *Obesity Research,* 10 (2002): 78–82.

Jenkins, D.J., T.M. Wolever, V. Vuksan, et al. "Nibbling versus gorging: Metabolic advantages of increased meal frequency." *New England Journal of Medicine,* 321 (1989): 929–34.

Mela, D.J. "Determinants of food choice: Relationships with obesity and weight control." *Obesity Research,* 9 (2001): S249–55.

Nielsen, S.J., et al. "Trends in energy intake in U.S. between 1977 and 1996: Similar shifts seen across age groups." *Obesity Research,* 10 (2002): 370–78.

Sparti, A., et al. "Effect of diets high or low in unavailable and slowly digestible carbohydrates on the pattern of 24-h substrate oxidation and feelings of hunger in humans." *American Journal of Clinical Nutrition,* 72 (2000): 1461–68.

Hu, F.B., et al. "Television watching and other sedentary behaviors in relation to risk of obesity and type 2 diabetes mellitus in women." *Journal of the American Medical Association,* 289 (2003): 1785–91.

Story, M., and P. Faulkner. "The prime time diet: A content analysis of eating behavior and food messages in television program content and commercials." *American Journal of Public Health,* 80 (1990): 738–40.

Robinson, T.N. "Reducing children's television viewing to prevent obesity, a randomized controlled trial." *Journal of the American Medical Association,* 282 (1999): 1561–67.

Bellisle, F., et al. "Cognitive restraint can be offset by distraction, leading to increased meal intake in women." *American Journal of Clinical Nutrition,* 74 (2001): 197–200.

Oliver, G., et al. "Stress and food choice: A laboratory study." *Psychosomatic Medicine,* 62 (2000): 853–65.

## 14: Lifestyle

Nielsen, S.J., et al. "Trends in energy intake in U.S. between 1977 and 1996: Similar shifts seen across age groups." *Obesity Research*, 10 (2002): 370–78.

# INDEX